Short Notes for Dental PG Entrance Examinations

Second Edition

Including Review for UG Students

Basic Sciences Volume 2

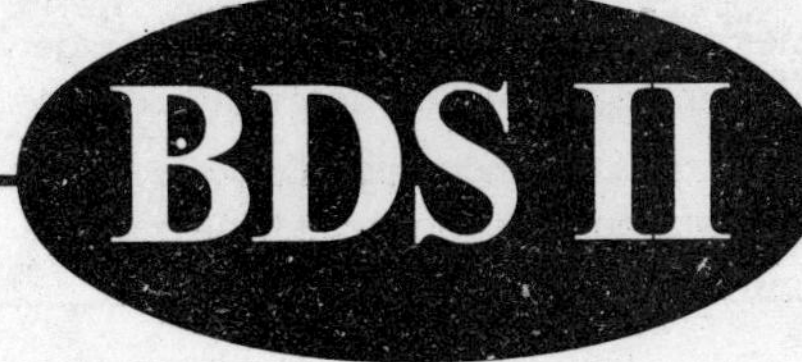

Volumes in the Series

Short Notes for **Dental PG Entrance Examinations**

Second Edition

Basic Sciences

- **Volume 1** BDS I
- **Volume 2** BDS II
- **Volume 3** BDS III

Clinical Sciences

- **Volume 4** Operative Dentistry, Endodontics, Oral Surgery, Local Anaesthesia, Orthodontics, Pedodontics
- **Volume 5** Periodontics, Prosthodontics, Basic Radiology Self-Assessment Paper, Model Test Papers

Short Notes for Dental PG Entrance Examinations

Second Edition

Including Review for UG Students

Basic Sciences Volume 2

SANDEEP GOYAL MDS (Orthodontics)
Professor
Department of Orthodontics and Dentofacial Orthopedics
ITS College of Dental Sciences and Research
Murad Nagar, UP

Edited by
Sonia Goyal MDS (Oral and Maxillofacial Surgery)
Associate Professor, Department of Oral and Maxillofacial Surgery,
ITS College of Dental Sciences and Research, Murad Nagar, UP

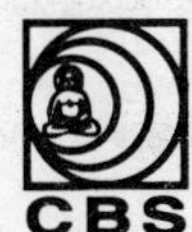

CBS Publishers & Distributors Pvt Ltd

New Delhi • Bangalore • Pune • Cochin • Chennai

Second Edition

Short Notes for Dental PG Entrance Examinations

Volume 2

First Edition : 2004
Second Edition : 2010

ISBN : 978-81-239-1799-3

Published by Satish Kumar Jain and produced by Vinod K. Jain for
CBS Publishers & Distributors Pvt Ltd
4819/XI Prahlad Street, 24 Ansari Road, Daryaganj,
New Delhi 110 002, India.
Fax: 011-23243014 e-mail: cbspubs@vsnl.com; delhi@cbspd.com
Website: www.cbspd.com

Branches

- **Bangalore:** Seema House 2975, 17th Cross, K.R. Road, Banasankari 2nd Stage, Bangalore 560 070
  Fax: 080-26771680 e-mail: cbsbng@gmail.com
- **Pune:** Shaan Brahmha Complex, Basement, Appa Balwant Chowk,
  Budhwar Peth, next to Ratan Talkies, Pune 411 002
  Fax: 020-24464059 e-mail: pune@cbspd.com
- **Cochin:** 36/14 Kalluvilakam, Lissie Hospital Road, Cochin-682018, Kerala.
  e-mail: cochin@cbspd.com
- **Chennai:** 20, West Park Road, Shenoy Nagar, Chennai 600030.
  email: chennai@cbspd.com

Printed at Somya Printers, Delhi-110053

dedicated
to
Ma Vaishno Devi,
my parents
and
my teachers

Acknowledgments

At the very outset, I bow my head to the Almighty God and my Guruji for all the grace showered on me to compile the second edition of the book. I am also thankful to my parents for their unforgettable sacrifices and choicest blessings.

I acknowledge the words of advice given to me by Dr Prof. Hari Parkash, Director General, ITS College of Dental Sciences and Research, Murad Nagar.

I place on record my deep gratitude towards my mentors and guides, my respected teachers during my postgraduation, Dr D N Kapoor, the then Professor and Head; Dr V P Sharma, Professor; Dr Pradeep Tandon, Professor, Department of Orthodontics and Dentofacial Orthopedics, Faculty of Dental Sciences, KGMC, Lucknow, for all their blessings, ideas and inspiration.

Prof P B Sood, Principal, ITS College of Dental Sciences and Research, Murad Nagar, has always been a constant source of insipiration and advice.

Dr Sanjay Tiwari, Professor and Head, Department of Endodontics, and Principal, GDC, PGIMS, Rohtak, for all his good wishes, the support, stimulating criticism and magnanimous help during my UG/PG days and afterwards.

My wife Dr Sonia Goyal MDS (oral and maxillofacial surgery), for her support, constant advice, contribution and editing the text, and all the pains she took during the compilation of the project.

Mr S K Jain and Mr Y N Arjuna of CBS Publishers & Distributors Pvt Ltd and their team of professionals for their best suggestions and help in getting this work published in the present form.

Last but not the least, I acknowledge all my family members and friends for their best wishes to boost my morale.

Sandeep Goyal MDS

Preface to the Second Edition

We thank all our readers for their overwhelming support and inputs for the first edition of our series **Short Notes for PG Dental Entrance Examinations**. However, with the increasing competition and increasing base of knowledge, a strong requirement for the improvement has been felt.

In the second edition, we have tried to incorporate a few new topics which will be helpful to postgraduate aspirants. We have now compiled the basic subjects and clinical subjects separately. This will help those undergraduate students also who aspire to compete for postgraduate entrance examination in the future. This edition will help and guide them to build their knowledge base from the very beginning of their dental career and will be helpful in their regular BDS examinations and also *viva voce* examinations.

We have included MCQs in this new edition for the side-by-side exercise and testing the skills and growth of their knowledge base. The book in the second edition has now been split into five volumes, considering the valuable additions made in the text as well new sections of MCQs which have been selectively added to strengthen the inherent appeal of this title amongst the potential readers. Basic Sciences are covered in Vols 1–3 and Clinical Sciences in Vols 4 and 5.

We request our readers to continue sending their suggestions to us for future improvements for the benefit of their friends, juniors and other future dental surgeons.

In the end, we again emphasize that all the aspirants should synergize their knowledge by reading standard theory books to smoothly sail through the ocean of entrance examination, since our volumes may not be complete in every aspect.

Sandeep Goyal MDS
Sonia Goyal MDS
goyalsandeep2000@rediffmail.com
goyalsandeep2000@gmail.com

Preface to the First Edition

There has been a marked increase in competition in dental PG entrance examinations, which have become tougher in recent times. A proper guidance to the aspirants is, therefore, necessary for making their preparations.

The trend of today being MCQ-based, the aspirants just memorise the MCQs from the books available in the market without going into the depth of the statement, leading to errors during the examination. Also, a series of MCQs currently available in the market unfortunately contain 50 to 60% repetition of the questions, and the answers to many questions given in the answer key are also misleading and confusing for the students.

Most of the students do not want to undertake a detailed study of the subjects for their preparation and hence look for the easiest method to get through in the examinations which they consider to be present in the MCQ books.

In my view, MCQ books are for practice only. Your basic knowledge is tested through MCQs and they help to churn your mind, but you should not read them blindly thinking that they will be repeated in the examinations as such. The paper setters change the statements and options of the MCQs for better judgement of the student, therefore, only those students who have a strong basic knowledge can easily analyze and correlate the statement and the option. Also, for some of those students who read the textbooks and do not make notes but rather underline the text or write in the textbooks only, revision becomes very confusing and time-consuming.

This book has been compiled with an idea in mind to provide handy information in the form of a ready-reckoner to the aspirants. This volume covers eight important subjects, and other subjects will be included in the latter volume(s). The motive of compiling information in this manner is to bring important points of each topic together so that a student while reading the topics can revise all the key points immediately and at one stretch.

I have tried with the best possible efforts to tabulate and alphabetically arrange most of the important information so as to make it easy for the students to search for the required topic. The book speaks about the points to be stressed in the form of lists, like the most common terms, syndromes, synonyms, etc.

This book gives the students the guidelines and information about the topics most often asked in the examinations. However, they are advised to go for **further detailed reading from standard textbooks to supplement and reinforce their knowledge.**

I have attempted my best to include almost 80 to 90% of the important information on the covered subjects. However, the readers must study additionally and add their own points on the topics for their benefit.

No project can be completed and improved upon without **feedback**, constructive criticism and healthy suggestions. It is my humble request to all the readers and students to send me their suggestions and points/topics to be added in further editions of the book, to make it more informative and useful for their younger friends and students. It is promised that these suggestions will be suitably incorporated in the future editions and all the contributors will be suitably acknowledged. My e–mail address is goyalsandeep2000@sify.com. Wishing you all the success in your examinations.

Sandeep Goyal MDS

Suggested Readings

Since we do not claim this book to be complete in all the respects, we advise the students to further supplement their information by going through other standard textbooks on particular topics. We are providing below a list of some books for reference for the students.

	Author	Textbook on
1.	Monheim's	Local anesthesia
2.	Malamed's	Local anesthesia
3.	Graber's	Orthodontics – an art or science
4.	Profitt's	Orthodontics
5.	Grossman's	Endodontics
6.	Cohen's	Endodontics, i.e. pathways to the pulp
7.	Ingle's	Endodontics
8.	Gupta	Removable Partial Prosthodontics
9.	Orban's	Dental and oral histology
10.	Ten cate's	Oral histology
11.	Shafer's	Oral pathology
12.	Stone's	Oral pathology
13.	Burkitt's	Oral medicine
14.	Sikri	Dental Radiology, 4/e
15.	Sikri	Conservative Dentistry
16.	Goaz /White	Radiology
17.	Singh	Embryology
18.	Garg	Histology, 4/e

Standard books of MCQs which should be read definitely:

- Series of NDBs, i.e. national dental board papers, available upto L – series in I and II volumes.
- Rudman's
- Boucher's
- Steele's
- Gardiner's
- Cawson's
- Reed's Vols I & II
- Arco's Vols I & II

Besides these books, the students should always refer to the MCQ books available in the market for practice but they should not get confused.

Contents of Volume 2

Contents of Volumes 1 and 3

VOLUME 1 BDS I

VOLUME 3 BDS III

Abbreviations Used in the Book

- AD — autosomal dominant
- A. — artery
- Ag/Ab/ — antigen/antibody
- Aka — also known as
- Alv. — alveolar
- Ant./post. — anterior/posterior
- As — arsenic
- Ass. — associated
- B/W — between
- Bact. — bacteria
- BCC — basal cell ca.
- C/E — clinical exam.
- Ca. — carcinoma
- Ch. — chronic/characteristics
- Chr. — chromosomes
- Cp. — compared
- CT — connective tissue
- Def. — deficiency
- Dev. — develop/developmental
- Dis — disease/distance as per the case
- D/D — differential diagnosis
- Enz. — enzyme
- Epith. — epithelium/-al
- ECA/ICA — external/internal carotid A
- H/E — histology examination
- IU — intrauterine
- LAP — lymphadenopathy
- LN — lymph nodes
- LO — lateral oblique
- M. — muscles
- Mm — mucous membrane
- MO/m.o. — malocclusion
- Md/mand — mandibular
- Memb. — membrane
- MNGC — multinucleated giant cells
- MNP/LNP — median/lateral nasal process

❑ Mo.	months
❑ Mx/max	maxillary
❑ n.m.	neuromuscular
❑ O/F	oral features
❑ Org./orgs.	organisms
❑ OTM	orthodontic tooth movement
❑ OMV	occipito-mental view
❑ OFD	object – film dis.
❑ PO	presence of
❑ PA	periapical/posteroanterior
❑ PNS	para nasal sinus
❑ Pt.	patient
❑ PDL	periodontal ligament
❑ R/G	radiograph
❑ R/L	radiolucent
❑ R/O	radiopaque
❑ REE	reduced enamel epith
❑ Reqd.	required
❑ SCC	squamous cell ca.
❑ SG	salivary gland
❑ S/S	signs and symptoms
❑ SMV	submento-vertex view
❑ Synd	syndrome
❑ TFD	target-film distance
❑ TOD	target – object dis.
❑ Vit.	vitamin

How to Prepare for the Entrance Examinations

This is my personal experience for PG entrance preparation and a time-tested method as many of my friends who have followed this method have been successful in the exams.

1. You have to believe in that hard work and luck go side by side.
2. Keep at least 6–8 months for preparation, which should be free from any sort of disturbance and forget about your surroundings.
3. Devote at least 8–10 hrs/day for the studies.
4. Divide your time and make a time bound schedule.
5. Pick important subjects first depending on the numbers of questions asked in the examinations. The subjects to be studied and stressed during entrance preparation are : general anatomy; dental materials; dental histology; pharmacology; oral pathology; fluorides; endodontics; periodontology; local anaesthesia; pedodontics; basics of all the clinical subjects.
6. Make your daily routine and diligently follow it.
7. Read MCQs two times from NDBs and any other standard book available on a particular subject. This will give you an idea about the style of MCQs and the part of the topic from which the question has been picked from the text, e.g. many MCQs are taken from the legends written below the figures in the book especially dental histology, periodontology, orthodontics.
8. Pick up a standard textbook which you have read during UG days. Read the topics and make notes separately and underline the important points. This will help you to strengthen your knowledge on that topic. Then take other subjects and follow the same pattern.
9. Read only relevant parts of the non-clinical subjects. Stress on anatomy, embryology, dental histology, pharmacology and physiology during the preparation.

10. All the topics and subjects should be covered in the time that at least two months are left for revision before the examination which you are preparing for.
11. When you have finished all the subjects, pick the MCQs books and read the 2–3 times. Any problem can be referred to your notes/textbooks.
12. Mark difficult MCQs in the book with different colors and read them carefully everytime.
13. 15 days before exams, read the notes on all the subjects, followed by one more revision of MCQs.
14. Discussion with your friends is a very important part of preparation. It gives an insight into the topics and more informations.
15. Take all the exams as far as possible; it tells you the trend; your standing and reshuffles your knowledge.

If you follow these rules, I can guarantee you 100% success in the examinations.

Syllabus

Given below is brief outline of the syllabus and topics the students should follow during preparation which should be supplemented by other topics for better knowledge.

Subjects	Topics	Books advised
Anatomy	♦ Head and neck — complete ♦ Brain — basics	Chaurasia's
Embryology	♦ Basics ♦ Pharyngeal arches ♦ Fetal circulation ♦ Fate of germ layers ♦ Development of oral cavity and face	I B Singh
Histology	♦ Basics ♦ Cell structure, cell division ♦ All glands and appendages, spleen, liver, etc. ♦ Skin, epithelium, A, V, N, M, CT	I B Singh
Dental materials	Complete	Skinners
Physiology	♦ Basics ♦ Blood, GIT, CVS, respiration, endocrinology	Chatterjee
Biochemistry	Basic concepts, enzymes, DNA/RNA, Krebs's cycle, HMP, etc. cycles carbohydrate/ lipid/ protein structure and metabolism, vitamins, minerals, energy requirements, etc.	Rama Rao, Harper's

Subjects	**Topics**	**Books advised**
Dental histology	Complete	Orbans
Dental anatomy	Basics, difference in morphology of molars, premolars, canines, mand lateral incisors, etc., occlusion, TMJ, alveolar bone	Wheeler's
Microbiology	Basics, sterilisation, structure of bacteria and virus, immunity, Ag–Ab reactions, *Strept.*, *Staph., Clostridia, Mycobacterium,* HIV, Hepatitis virus	Ananthnarayan
Pathology	Basics only, neoplasia definitions, blood pathology (Do not waste much time on it.)	Robins
Pharmacology	Basic concepts, pharmacokinetics and dynamics, dental pharmacology, antibiotics, analgesics, LA/GA, sympathomimetic/lytic drugs, cholinergics/adrenergic, etc., briefly about CVS, CNS, antiepileptic, etc. Mechanism of action of all the drugs, MCQs	K D Tripathi
Oral pathology	Complete	Shafer's
Surgery/ medicine	Basics only, HT, TB, DM, infections, etc.	Any book
PCD	Fluorides, epidemiology, definitions, indices;	
Orthodontics	Basics, growth, ceph, diagnosis, appliances, wire properties, tissue reactions, forces, anchorage, tooth movements	Graber's, Proffit's

Subjects	Topics	Books advised
Local anesthesia	Complete	Monheim's, Malamed
Oral surgery	Basics; sterilisation, sutures, grafts, fascial infections, maxillary sinus, TMJ, salivary glands, fractures and x-rays	Kruger's, Killey's
Operative	Basics, cavity preparation, classification, cariolgy, instruments, cements and restorative materials, differences between cavity of silver, gold, porcelain, etc.	Sturdevant, Marzouk
Endodontics	Complete book	Grossman, Weine
Pedodontics	Complete book	Mcdonald's, Finn's
Periodontics	Complete book	Glickmann's
Radiography	Brief, basics	Any standard book
Prosthodontics	Basics of CD/impressions; materials, occlusions, jaw relations, implants, TMJ, movements, immediate dentures, etc. Basics of FPD preparations, finish lines, crown preparations, principles, gingival retraction, impression, casting, etc. Basics of RPD, DR, IR, connectors, classification of RPDs, diagnosis and Rx plan, surveyor, etc.	Boucher's Fenn Winkler's Shillinburg Dykema McCracken's Steward

BDS II

10

Dental Anatomy

NOMENCLATURE

(1) **Universal system** =

(a) for primary teeth.

ABCDE	FGHIJ
TSRQP	ONMLK

(b) For permanent teeth =

1,2,3,4,5,6,7,8	9,10,11,12,13,14,15,16
32,31,30,29,28,27,26,25,	24,23,22,21,20,19,18,17

(2) **palmar notation** = it uses quadrant system, but incompatible to computers etc.; aka ZSIG MONDY system; it is the oldest system.

(a) For deciduous teeth =

EDCBA	ABCDE
EDCBA	ABCDE

(b) For permanent teeth =

87654321	12345678
87654321	12345678

(3) **FDI / WHO notation** = it is a 2-digit system, (1971)

(a) For permanent teeth

18,17,16,15,14,13,12,11	21,22,23,24,25,26,27,28
48,47,46,45,44,43,42,41	31,32,33,34,35,36,37,38

(b) For deciduous teeth =

55,54,53,52,51	61,62,63,64,65
85,84,83,82,81	71,72,73,74,75

BASIC POINTS

- Main bulk of tooth is composed of = **dentin** (ie root and crown).
- Part of pulp cavity present in crown part of tooth is ka = pulp chamber.
- Soft tissue of tooth = pulp.
- Hard tissue of tooth = enamel, dentin, cementum (C,D,E).
- Alveolar process = part of jaw which serves as a support for the tooth.
- Only 4 teeth have their mesial surfaces in contact with each other are = central incisors.
- Cusp = is an elevation on the crown as a divisional part of occlusal surface.
- Tubercle = is a **deviation**; is a smaller elevation on some portion of crown produced by an extra formation of enamel. Present on max 1; mand 4; max 6.
- Cingulum = lingual lobe of anterior tooth and makes the bulk of cervical 3rd of lingual surface.
- Triangular ridge = descends from the tips of the cusp of molars / premolars towards the central part of occlusal surface; **relate to one cusp only.**
- Transverse ridge = when the triangular ridges of buccal and lingual cusp join and cross transversely the surface of a posterior tooth. It is present on pri. mand. D and permanent max 6; and mand 4.
- **Oblique ridge** = on maxillary molars only; formed by the union of triangular ridge of DB cusp and distal cusp ridge of ML cusp.
- Triangular fossa = on molars / premolars on occlusal surface, mesial or distal to the marginal ridges.
- Sulcus = is a long depression / valley b/w ridges and cusps.
- Groove = line / groove b/w the primary parts of crown or root.
- Pits = located at the junction / terminals of developmental grooves.
- Lobes = is one of the primary sections of formation in the development of crown, e.g. cusp, memelons.
- Memelons = present on the incisal ridge of newly erupted incisor teeth.

- Line angles of anterior tooth = 6
- Line angles of posterior tooth = 8
- Point angles of anterior tooth = 4
- Point angles of posterior tooth = 4

Table of MD tooth dimension

Tooth	Max.	Mand.
1	8.5 mm	5.0 mm
2	6.5	5.5
3	7.5	7.0
4	7.0	7.0
5	7.0	7.0
6	10.0	11.0
7	9.0	10.5
8	8.5	10.0

Table of chronology: permanent teeth

Teeth	First evidence of calcification	Crown completed (yrs.)	Eruption (yrs.)	Root completed (yrs.)
Maxillary				
1	3–4mo	4–5	7–8	10
2	10–12 mo	4–5	8–9	11
3	4–5 mo	6–7	11–12	13–15
4	1 ½ -1 ¾ years	5–6	10–11	12–13
5	2–2 ¼ years	6–7	10–12	12–14
6	At birth	2 ½–3	6–7	9–10
7	2 ½-3 years	7–8	12–13	14–16
8	7–9 years	12–16	17–21	18–25

Table of chronology: permanent teeth (*Contd.*)

Mandible				
1	3–4 mos	4–5 years	6–7 years	9 years
2	3–4 mos	4–5	7–8	10
3	4–5 mos	6–7	9–10	12–14
4	1 ¾–2 years	5–6	10–12	12–13
5	2 ¼–2 ½, show variations	6–7	11–12	13–14
6	At birth	2½–3	6–7	9–10
7	2 ½–3 years	7–8	11–13	14–15
8	8–10	12–16	17–21	18–25

Chronology of primary teeth

Teeth	**1st evidence of calcification**	**Crown completed**	**Eruption**	**Root completed**
Maxillary A	14 wk i.u	1½ mos.	10 mos	1½ years
B	16	2½	11	2
C	17	9	19	3¼
D	15 ½	6	16	2½
E	19	11	29	3
Mandibular A	14	2½	8	1½
B	16	3	13	1½
C	17	9	20	3¼
D	15 ½	5 ½	16	2¼
E	18	10	27	3

- Crown completion of pri dentition = 12 months
- Crown completion of permanent dentition = 8 yrs
- Root end completed of pri dentition = 3 yrs
- Root end completed of permanent dentition = 16 yrs; except 3rd molars
- Root end completed of 3rd molars = 18 – 25 yrs
- Sequence of eruption of pri teeth = ABDCE
- A = 6–8 mos
- B = 8–10 mos
- C = 16–20 mos
- D = 12–16 mos
- E = 20–30 mos

Amount of enamel formed in primary teeth at birth

TEETH	In maxillary	In mandibular
CI	5/6th	3/5th
LI	2/3rd	3/5th
CANINE	1/3rd	1/3rd
1ST Molar	**Cusps united**; occlusal completely calcified + a ½ to 3/4th crown height	**Cusps united**; occlusal completely calcified.
2ND Molar	Cusps united; occlusal incompletely calcified; calcified tissue on a 5th to a 4th crown height.	Cusps united; occlusal incompletely calcified.

Nolla's stages of tooth calcification: it is divided into 10 stages as follows

- 0 absence of crypt
- 1 **presence of crypt**
- 2 initial calcification

- 3 — 1/3rd of the crown completed
- 4 — 2/3rd of the crown completed
- 5 — crown almost completed
- 6 — **crown completed**
- 7 — 1/3rd of root completed
- 8 — 2/3rd of root completed
- 9 — root almost completed; **open apex**
- 10 — apical end of **root completed**

Eruption = i.e. continuous tooth movement from dental bud to occlusal contact.

Emergence = i.e. tooth emerging through the gingiva.

Dental age = i.e. based on the no. of teeth erupted or on stages of the development of teeth / root development etc.

Chronological age = i.e. from the birth day.

Skeletal age = i.e. from the bones development stages.

Chronologies of the eruption of teeth are less satisfactory (due to caries, tooth loss, etc.) for dental age assessment than those based on tooth formation.

Age attainment schedules = are useful clinically where it is necessary to avoid damage to developing teeth during treatment.

Age prediction chronology = for assessing unknown ages of the patients and for forensic purpose.

PRIMARY DENTITION

- Calcification of primary teeth starts at = 13 – 16 wks i.u. (First trimester)
- All primary teeth begin to calcify at = 18 – 20 wks i.u. (2nd trimester)
- Emergence of primary teeth occur b/w = 6 – 30 mos. age.
- Primary dentition to be completed requires = 2 – 3 years beginning with initial calcification of primary incisors to the completion of roots of 2nd molars.

- Each permanent tooth takes 8 – 14 years to complete if 3rd molar is considered.
- Eruption sequence = ABDCE; in it D and mandibular E show sexual difference also.
- BDC tend to erupt earlier in maxilla than mandible.
- Premature loss of primary teeth from dental neglect = causes loss of arch length / crowding of primary teeth.

PERMANENT DENTITION

Formation of teeth occurs in **clusters** as

1. **First cluster** = 6123 = formation begins in 1st year
2. **Second cluster** = formation begins in 2 – 4 years
3. **Third cluster** = 3rd molar = formation begins 5 – 6 years after 2nd molar.

First molar = first permanent tooth to erupt; ka 6 year molar; **begins to calcify at birth**.

2nd molar = aka 12 year molar

3rd molar = aka 18 year molar; wisdom tooth.

Eruption sequence = 61245378 or 61243578 in upper arch; 61234578 in lower arch.

Mandibular permanent teeth erupt before maxillary teeth.

Follicles of permanent 123 are = lingual to primary teeth roots.

Premolars = lie within the bifurcation of primary molar roots.

1 – 5 teeth = aka **succedaneous teeth**, as they have primary predecessors also.

More than 6 months delay in eruption of a tooth from its average age of eruption means DELAYED ERUPTION.

DEVELOPMENT OF TEETH

- **4 or more centers of formation** of each tooth.
- **Minimum No. of developmental lobes** required for formation of permanent tooth = 4
- Each cusp is ka lobe.

- Separated by developmental grooves.
- Root formation is **approx half finished** = when the tooth emerges in the oral cavity.
- **Time required for root completion** after eruption = 2 – 3 years.
- Dental pulp = its primary function is to form dentin of the tooth.
- Pulp size is larger in = primary and young permanent teeth
- Protection of pulp by secondary dentin; dentin keeps on forming throughout life but at a slower rate. (Refer to section on dental histology in volume I.)

PRIMARY TEETH

- Are 20 in no.
- Period of stability is very short.
- Upper and lower E's and upper A are most unstable teeth.
- Eruption is ABDCE; mandibular erupt faster than maxillary.
- High peak of caries attack = approx at 13 years age
- Exfoliation of primary teeth b/w = 7th – 12th year of age
- Root resorption of primary teeth starts at = 1 – 2 years after complete root formation and apical foramen established.
- Needed for many years of growth and physical development and for space maintenance for permanent teeth.
- Primary dentition is complete at approx = 2 ½ years of age.
- Normal features = upright incisors; spacing ; attrition
- There are no teeth in deciduous set which resemble the premolars; maxillary D crown resembles maxillary 4,5 and permanent molars but may have 3 roots.
- **Mandibular D is unique** as = it has a crown form unlike that of any permanent tooth, but has 2 roots, i.e. M and D.
- Crowns of maxillary and mandibular Ds differ from any teeth in permanent set.
- No fluorosis is seen in primary teeth.

Difference b/w primary and permanent teeth: primary teeth are

- Narrower at neck; narrower occlusal surfaces;
- Prominent cervical ridges esp buccal of Ds.

- Roots flared widely; for p.o. permanent teeth in b/w roots.
- Primary anterior teeth crown have = MD > crown length (as cp to permanent teeth).
- Cervical ridges buccally on primary molars are much pronounced esp on D/D.
- High pulp horns and larger pulp chambers esp MESIAL HORN.
- Greater thickness of dentin over the pulpal wall at the occlusal fossa of primary molars.
- **Enamel rods** at CEJ **slope occlusally or are horizontal,** instead of gingivally / apically in permanent teeth.

Morphology of teeth

DECIDUOUS MAXILLARY CENTRAL INCISORS

1. MD dim > crown length (opposite in permanent maxillary C.I)
2. Cingulum extends up towards the incisal ridge to make a partial division of concavity on the lingual surface below the incisal edge, practically dividing it in a M and D fossa.

DECIDUOUS MAXILLARY LATERAL INCISORS

1. Crown length > MD width (as cp. to A)
2. DI angle of crown is more rounded.
3. Ratio of root / crown length > DECIDUOUS MAXILLARY CENTRAL INCISORS.

DECIDUOUS MAXILLARY CANINE

1. M and D contact areas are at the same level (as cp to permanent maxillary canine).
2. Mesial slope of cusp > distal slope (as cp to permanent canine).
3. Tip of cusp is distal to center of crown to allow for intercuspation with mandibular C; (which has D > M slope)

DECIDUOUS MANDIBULAR CENTRAL INCISORS

1. Resembles mandibular permanent LI
2. Root is = approx 2 x crown length

3. Its labio-lingual dimension is only approx 1 mm less than DECIDUOUS MAXILLARY CENTRAL INCISOR.

DECIDUOUS MANDIBULAR LATERAL INCISORS

1. Larger in all dimensions than mandibular A except labiolingual
2. Incisal ridge slopes downwards distally – s t distal contact area is apical for proper contact with mesial of mandibular C.

DECIDUOUS MANDIBULAR CANINE

- Thicker at the neck of the tooth as cp to maxillary C.
- Maxillary C is much larger labiolingually than mandibular C.
- Distal cusp slope > mesial (as cp to maxillary C)

DECIDUOUS MAXILLARY FIRST MOLAR

- 3 roots; Distal root < mesial root < lingual root (largest).
- bifurcation begins almost immediately at the site of the CEJ.
- ML cusp = most prominent; *longest*; sharpest
- DL cusp = poorly defined
- From mesial aspect, the dimensions at cervical 3rd are > at occlusal 3rd; ML cusp > MB cusp.
- A **prominent convexity on buccal outline is an outstanding feature** of this tooth which is an overdevelopment in this area; it does not continue distally.
- Crown tapers towards distal surface.
- DB cusp > DL cusp
- Crown outline **converges LINGUALLY and distally.**
- Oblique ridge = from ML – DB cusp.
- **Crown of maxillary D resembles permanent maxillary PMs**.
- DMR size << MMR in development (marginal ridge).

DECIDUOUS MAXILLARY 2ND MOLAR

- Resembles maxillary 6.
- 2 buccal cusps = nearly of same size

- 3 lingual cusps = ML > DL > supplemental cusp (which is apical to ML cusp and ka 5th cusp or **tubercle of Carabelli**).
- 3 roots = L > M > D
- ML > MB cusp
- From mesial aspect = MB root is very wide and forms 2/3rd the width of root trunk.
- Point of bifurcation b/w DB root and lingual root is more apical in location than any of the other points of bifurcation and it is in the center of crown on distal aspect (than on mesial aspect).
- Oblique ridge = from ML – DB cusp.
- Distal surface < mesial surface = crown **converges DISTALLY**.
- DMR = MMR in size (cp. to max. D)

DECIDUOUS MANDIBULAR FIRST MOLAR

- **Does not resemble any of the other teeth**, i.e. primary / permanent.
- Mesial surface is almost straight from contact area to CEJ = so CONSTRICTING THE CROWN VERY LITTLE AT THE CEJ.
- Distal part of crown is shorter than mesial part, so **cervical line** DIPS APICALLY where it joins the mesial root.
- It looks **like the fusion of 2 teeth**, the mesial half is 2 X taller than the distal half and mesial root is taller than the distal root.
- Crown converges LINGUALLY; but **spreads / widens DISTALLY** (as cp. to max. D).
- ML cusp is longest = is an **outstanding feature** and is centered lingually in line with mesial root.
- MB crown length is > ML, so **CEJ slants upwards** bucco-lingually.
- ML cusp is the largest cusp.
- It is the only tooth which widens DISTALLY.

DECIDUOUS MANDIBULAR 2 ND MOLAR

- Resembles mandibular 6 (crown of E is narrow buccolingually than MD than is in mandibular 6).

- Narrow at the cervical part (mandibular 6 is wider).
- Buccal surface equally divided in 3 cusps, i.e. MB, buccal , DB (mandibular 6 has 3 unequal cusps).
- **Crown narrows / converges lingually; and distally**.
- Crown extends out over the root more distally than it does mesially.
- Crown is **tipped distally**, i.e. mesial part is higher than the distal.
- MMR is high and so MB and ML cusps appear short from mesial aspect.

OCCLUSION OF PRIMARY TEETH

- Outline of upper teeth in arch = ellipse
- Except maxillary E and mandibular A, all other teeth occlude with 2 teeth of the opposing jaw.
- Roots of all primary teeth fully formed = at 3 years of age
- Diastema develop with growth after = 1 year or so after full eruption of teeth, i.e. approx 3 + years.
- In anteriors = permanent teeth come from LINGUAL side of primary teeth; it leads to spacing b/w teeth at 4 – 5 years of age.
- Severe attrition of teeth occurs during this phase; it helps in growth of mandible anteriorly, by removal occlusal interferences.
- Maxillary D occludes in MMR and mesial triangular fossa of mandibular E and distal 2/3rd of mandibular D.

PERMANENT TEETH

- Primary function of teeth = to prepare food for swallowing and to facilitate digestion.
- Human dentition is = **omnivorous**
- **Negative feedback** from receptors in PDL mediate the chewing forces ; Receptor threshold for axial forces is > than the tangential forces.
- Normally, the gingiva covers cervical 3rd of crown, ka Gingival line; it has got variable level.

- Cervical line is = STATIC anatomic landmark, i.e. CEJ
- **Curve of Spee** = is a segment of a sphere, in 3-dimensions.
- **Curve of Wilson** = lingual inclination of mandibular molars, i.e. concave for mandibular; convex for maxillary.
- Occlusal surfaces of maxillary molars make an acute angle mesially with long axis of its roots.

COMPARATIVE ANATOMY: 4 stages of tooth development / evolution

- Reptilian, i.e. **haplodont**
- Early mammalian, i.e. **triconodont**
- Triangular, i.e. **tritubercular molars**
- **Quadritubercular** molar

Reptilian stage

- Simplest, single cone
- Limit the jaw movements
- No occlusion
- Simple hinge movement

Triconodont stage

- 3 cusps in a LINE
- largest / main cusp is in the center.
- Anterior teeth = reflect the single cone
- Posterior teeth = 2 or more cones are fused.
- Each crown is a combination of 4 or more lobes.
- Anteriors = 3 labial lobes + 1 lingual lobe; labial lobes form the mamelons which are separated by labial grooves esp on maxillary 1; lingual lobe represent the cingulum.
- Tip of each cusp represents the **primary center of formation** of each lobe.

TOOTH FORMS

- Primates are BUNODONT and *isognathus* with limited lateral movement.

- **Bunodont** means = tooth bearing conical cusps.
- With **selenodont** molars = more lateral movement and more anisognathic.
- Earliest and simplest jaw movement = opening and closing.
- All aspects of tooth crown except incisal / occlusal are of 3 configurations, i.e. TRIANGLE; TRAPEZOID; RHOMBOID.
- Facial and lingual surfaces of all teeth = trapezoid; with short side at CEJ; and long side at occlusal / incisal.
- Longest uneven side of *trapezoid* represents occlusal line.
- Each permanent tooth has **2 antagonists except** mandibular 1 and maxillary 8.
- Mesial and distal aspects of 1,2,3 teeth = triangle shape
- Mesial and distal aspects of maxillary PMs and M teeth = trapezoidal; **Longest uneven side represents base of crown instead of occlusal line**. So occlusal surface is constricted to make it self-cleansing and easy mastication.
- Mesial and distal aspects of mandibular posterior teeth = rhomboidal shape; occlusal surfaces narrower than cervical; crown inclined to LINGUAL SIDE on the root base; axes of teeth of U/L jaws are kept parallel.
- Measurement of cervical part of primary tooth is smaller than occlusal part when seen from buccal / lingual aspects only.

SUMMARY

SHAPE	TEETH	ASPECT
Triangle	U/L 1,2,3 , i.e. six teeth	Mesial ; distal
Trapezoid	1. Occlusal side longest; U/L 1,2,3 anteriors and all posterior teeth.	Buccal and lingual aspects
Trapezoid	Shortest side occlusal = all U posterior teeth	M and D aspect
Rhomboids	All mandibular posterior teeth	M and D aspect

Shape of occlusal surfaces;

- Square = mand 5
- Rhomboidal = max 6; max E
- Rectangular = max 7
- Hexagonal / trapezoidal / pentagonal = mand 6
- Hexagonal = max 4
- Triangle / wedge shape = proximal aspect of all anterior teeth
- Trapezoid = proximal aspects of all max post teeth; labial and lingual aspect of all ant. Teeth; buccal and lingual aspect of all post teeth;
- Rhomboids = proximal aspect of all mand post teeth.
- **Buccal convergence** is present in = permanent max 6 and mand 5, i.e. these teeth have more broader lingual surface than the buccal surface.

PHYSIOLOGICAL FORMS OF THE TEETH

CONTACT AREAS

- All teeth except last molars has 2 contacting members.
- Canine and 1st PM , both U and L, contact at points rather than areas when newly erupted ; as there is no attrition,
- 7, 8 are prevented from drifting distally = by their angulation of occlusal surface to the root and by the angle of direction of occlusal forces.

INTERDENTAL SPACES

- Triangular shape;
- There is normally a distance of 1–1.5 mm b/w enamel and alveolar bone, i.e. distance of CEJ from crest of alveolar bone is 1–1.5 mm seen in R/G.
- Proper space b/w roots in the bone is v. Imp, for proper blood supply,. anchorage etc.

EMBREASURES / SPILL WAYS

- For escape of food during mastication;
- Prevents food from being forced through the contact areas;

EMBREASURES / SPILL WAYS from incisal and occlusal aspect

- Anterior teeth have their contact Areas located centered labiolingually.
- Posterior teeth have contact Areas **slightly buccal to the center** buccolingually.
- Except maxillary 6, all crowns converge more lingually than facially from the contact areas.
- Maxillary 6 is the **only tooth wider lingually** than buccally, so ML embreasure is narrower/ smaller.

HEIGHT OF CONTOUR / HOC

HOC ON BUCCAL / LINGUAL SURFACES

- deflect the food away from gingival margins during mastication.
- Normal cervical curvature from CEJ to the crest of contour is approx 0.5 mm in extent.
- Crest of curvature/HOC on all posterior teeth on LINGUAL SIDE is at/near the middle 3rd of the crowns and is approx 1 mm.

HEIGHT OF EPITHELIAL ATTACHMENT

- EA seals the soft tissues to the tooth.
- Follows the CEJ curve and is higher than the CEJ.
- EA is highest at median line on central incisors; the height of EA decreases distally along with the CEJ curvatures till mesial surface of first PM. After this, to the 3rd molar, the curvature is slight.

PERMANENT TEETH

Maxillary 1 and mandibular 2

From incisal aspect, the ML > DL side, i.e. cingulum's center is towards the distal surface.

In the following teeth, the MD > BL dimensions, i.e. maxillary 1,2 and mandibular 6,7,8.

Cingulum of maxillary 2 and mandibular 1 is located in MD center of the crowns.

Differences b/w maxillary and mandibular 2 are : in mandibular 2 there are—

- A root groove / depression on distal surface of mandibular 2.
- Root of mandibular 2 is wider labiolingually than MD while of maxillary 2 is MD = BL dimension.
- Root of maxillary 2 is cone shaped and tapers towards lingual but of mandibular 2 is parallel.

Differences b/w mandibular 1 and mandibular 2 are: from the incisal aspect, the incisal edge is rotated (in accordance to the curvature of mandibular arch) on the root distolingually.

Maxillary 3 / canine

M < D slope = 3 (5 tooth PM_2)

M > D slope = 4 tooth (PM_1)

From labial aspect

- Outline of crown from CEJ to HOC mesially is convex and distally is concave.
- Cusp = mesial slope is < distal slope.

From mesial aspect: the cusp tip lies labial to the root tip as compared to maxillary 1,2 where tip and apex are in the same line.

From incisal aspect

- The **cusp is labial** to the center of crown labiolingually **and mesial** to the center of crown mesiodistally.
- BL thickness of crown on mesial > distal.

Mandibular 3 / canine: from labial aspect

- Mesial outline is nearly straight with mesial outline of the root.
- Mesial cusp ridge is < distal.

- Mesial contact area is towards incisal edge than distal CA.

From mesial aspect: cusp tip is more nearly centered over the root.

Maxillary 4 / PM 1

- **Mesial slope of cusp is > distal slope**, i.e. opposite of maxillary 3, so the tip of buccal cusp is distal to a line bisecting the buccal surface of the crown.
- Buccal HOC = is at the junction of cervical and middle 3rd.
- Tip of buccal cusp = directly below the tip of buccal root and is **nearer the center** of root trunk than of lingual cusp.
- Tip of lingual cusp = is on the line with the lingual border of lingual root.
- MMR = at the level of junction of middle and occlusal 3rd s.
- MESIAL DEVELOPMENTAL DEPRESSION = on mesial surface just below the contact area, it continues beyond CEJ and joins a deep developmental depression b/w the 2 roots.
- Well defined developmental groove in enamel of MMR which is a central groove on occlusal surface, immediately lingual to mesial CA (contact area).

From occlusal aspect = hexagonal shape; MB = DB; M < D; ML < DL dimensions.

Crest of distal CA is buccal to that of mesial

Crest of buccal ridge is DISTAL to that of lingual.

DB cusp ridge is BUCCAL to the MB cusp ridge.

Occlusal surface has NO SUPPLEMENTAL GROOVES.

MAXILLARY 5 / PM 2

Buccal aspect = mesial slope of buccal cusp is < distal (as cp to maxillary 4) (same as max. 3).

Mesial aspect = buccal and lingual cusps are of same height; (maxillary 4 has B > L cusp in height).

Distance b/w B and L cusp tip is more > in maxillary 4; so wider occlusal surface is there.

No developmental depression on mesial surface of crown (as is on maxillary 4)

No developmental groove crossing MMR.

Occlusal aspect = outline is rounded / oval; multilple supplementary grooves present; buccal cusp ridge of maxillary 5 is evenly convex.

Mandibular 4 / PM 1

MB cusp ridge < DB cusp ridge (ie same as mandibular 3)

M and D contact areas are nearly at same level.

Buccal aspect = MB < DB cusp ridges

Tip of buccal cusp = is located a little mesial to center of crown buccally.

Lingual aspect = crown tapers to LINGUAL side.

Major part made of middle buccal lobe.

Occlusal surface slopes greatly towards cervical direction.

MESIOLINGUAL DEVELOP GROOVE is an imp C/F (clinical feature) and is the line of demarcation b/w MB lobe and lingual lobe.

MESIAL ASPECT = rhomboidal outline;

Tip of buccal cusp nearly centered over the root tip

Lingual lobe's convexity is lingual to the root outline.

Crown tilted in lingual direction and so tip of lingual cusp is along the lingual outline of root (as cp to maxillary 4,5 which is within root trunk).

HOC on buccal aspect = in middle 3rd of crown.

Distal aspect = **DMR is higher than MMR** and does not have that extreme lingual slope as MMR has.

No developmental grooves as on MMR.

Occlusal aspect = smaller mesial CA in contact with mandibular 3 (due to ML developmental groove).

Mandibular 5/ PM 2

Buccal aspect = shorter height of cusps; MB and DB cusp ridges have lesser angulation than mandibular 4.

Lingual aspect = lingual lobes are more developed so cusps are longer / bulky.

Less of occlusal surface seen because the occlusal surface is not inclined lingually.

If 2 cusps = then ML > DL cusp, a groove b/w them centered on root. Groove is distal to center of the crown and **is Y-shaped.**

Size of PM 2 is > PM1.

Mesial aspect = as cp to mandibular 4 shows following differences–

- Buccal cusp not so nearly centered over the root trunk.
- Lingual lobe is developed more.
- Marginal ridges are at right angle to long axis of tooth
- No ML developmental-groove is there.

Distal aspect = more occlusal surface is seen as cp to mesial aspect because **DMR is at lower level than MMR.**

Crown of all posterior teeth are **tipped distally to long axis** of root of all the U / L teeth.

Occlusal aspect = if 2 cusps then round outline; if 3 cusps then square outline and Y – shape groove.

Maxillary 6 / M 1

Normal location of maxillary 6 is *at the center* of the fully developed adult jaw antero-posteriorly; it is ka CORNER STONE OF the dental arch. MB root is in line with KEY-RIDGE (of zygoma) in or normally positioned tooth; basis of angle's classification.

Crown width BL > MD by 1 mm.

Largest tooth in the maxillary arch.

4 major cusps = ML is largest / longest. Its MD width is 3/5th of the MD crown diameter. ML cusp lies on the long axis of lingual root. ML>MB>DL>DB>5th cusp.

fifth cusp = ka **cusp of Carabelli**; present on the ML surface of ML cusp; Lingual surface wider than buccal surface.

Point of root bifurcation is 4 mm from the CEJ.

PRIMARY CUSP TRIANGLE OF THE MAXILLARY MOLARS: according to the **Cope–Osborne theory of tooth origin** as the tritubercular stage in human tooth development, the **DL lobe becomes progressively smaller** from M1 to M3, rest of the area represents the primary cusp triangle.

Crown of this tooth tapers DISTALLY and buccally.

From occlusal aspect : rhomboidal shape; acute angles are MB / DL; obtuse angles are ML / DB.

Buccolingual dimension of mesial half is > on distal half.

MD dim immediate distal to contact area is > than the dimension mesial to contact area, i.e. CROWN WIDENS LINGUALLY AND MESIALLY, so the Lingual embreasure b/w 5,6 is narrow.

Oblique ridge = from DB to ML cusp.

2 major fossa = central and distal.

MAXILLARY. 7 / M 2

- No 5th cusp;
- Apex of lingual root is in line with DL cusp tip, instead of lingual groove as in maxillary 6.
- Crown converges distally.

Mandibular 6 / M 1

- Largest tooth of mandibular arch.
- MD dim > BL dim.

Buccal aspect = 3 cusps = MB > DB > distal

Height of lingual cusps is > buccal cusps.

From mesial aspect = BL dim of crown on mesial > distal, i.e. **crown converges DISTALLY**.

Entire crown has a **lingual tilt** i.r.t. the root axis.

Lingual cusp tips are within the lingual outline of the roots instead of being on a line with them.

Distal aspect = crown is *shorter distally* than mesially. Buccal and lingual surfaces **converge distally**.

Occlusal aspect = hexagonal;

MD > BL dim, i.e. **opposite of maxillary molars**

BL dim of crown on M > D

Crown converges LINGUALLY.

MB > ML = DL > DB > D cusps.

from a developmental point of view, all mandibular molars have 4 major cusps but all maxillary molars have 3 major cusps.

Mandibular 7 / M 2

4 cusps only, only one buccal development groove; while M 1 has 2 grooves. No distal cusp and DB groove.

PULP (Also refer to section on Dental Histology)

- Originate from mesenchyme.
- **Primary function** = formation of dentin
- Secondary dentin = is formed through out the life of tooth as a normal process, but it is not uniform b'coz odontoblasts adj to floor and roof of pulp cavity produce greater amounts of secondary dentin than adj to walls of pulp cavity.
- Reparative / irritation dentin = forms as a defensive response.
- Pulp within the pulp chamber is more cellular than in RC.
- Maxillary canine has largest labio-lingual root dim of any tooth of the mouth and so size of pulp chamber may also be the largest.
- Maxillary PM 1 = kidney shaped outline at cervical cross section with a *classic indentation* due to the mesial developmental groove.

MAXILLA = has 4 processes = zygomatic, palatine, frontal, alveolar bones.

Mandible = heaviest and strongest bone of head; mandibular fossa/ TMJ is in temporal bone.

Condyle = is wider mesiodistally than AP dimensions; its long axis is directed mesially and posteriorly.

Mental foramen (Refer section of Anatomy also)

- opening is directed U, B and laterally,
- in adults = is lies b/w roots of mandibular 4,5 below the apex.; midway b/w the upper and lower borders.
- In childhood = below mandibular D; nearer the lower border.
- After tooth loss = near the crest of alveolar border

Mandibular 7,8 are located 5 – 7 mm lingually to the anterior border of ramus.

A thin and perforated area of retromolar triangular space distal to M3 = is for rich blood supply and *cancellous bone*.

TEMPOROMANDIBULAR JOINT (Also refer section of Anatomy)

- Articular disc = collagenous; avascular; devoid of Ns in central area.
- **Condyle** = wider medio-laterally than AP by 2.5 x.; long axis directed posteriorly and medially, which meet at a point anterior to foramen magnum at an angle of 135.
- Mandibular fossa / articular eminence = is a part of squamous temporal bone.
- Mandibular fossa = divided in 2 halves, the anterior half is included in TMJ.
- Capsule = anterolateral side thickened to form TM – ligament; it arises on zygomatic arch; passes down and back to attach on the neck of mandible, main ligament of TMJ.
- Nerve supply of capsule = from 5th nerve;
- **Otomandibular lig**, e.g. disco-malleolar and tympano-mandibular/ sphenomandibular lig = which connect malleus to TMJ disc.
- Lateral ligament aka **TM lig** = is the main lig of TMJ.
- Articular disc = is avascular in the center. It has concavo-convex superior surface and concave inferior surface.
- **Articular disc** = a part of **superior head of lateral pterygoid** muscle inserts in disc and capsule. Relation of the disc to eminence is stabilised by upper head of lateral pterygoid m.

- Joint cavity is divided in 2 parts by the articular disc.
- **Upper compartment** = only gliding movement
- **Lower compartment** = both rotation and gliding movements.
- **Sphenomandibular ligament** = from spine of sphenoid and petrotympanic fissure to lingula of mandibular foramen; it is a **remnant of cephalic / dorsal end of Meckel's cartilage**. It is pierced by **mylohyoid Ns and vessels** at its lower end.
- **Stylomandibular lig.** = is thickened part of deep cervical fascia; it separates the parotid gland from the SMG. It runs from the styloid to the angle / posterior border of the ramus.
- Blood supply = by superficial temporal A and br of maxillary A.
- Nerve supply = by auriculotemporal N and masseteric N (Br. of 5th N)

MANDIBULAR POSITIONS

- CO / ICP = maximum intercuspation of teeth
- CR / RCP = in which condyles are in their uppermost midmost positions in the mandibular fossa and are related anteriorly to the distal slope of the articular eminence.
- CO is 1 mm anterior to CR, i.e. ka CO – CR discrepancy.
- CO = is a tooth determined position
- CR = is a jaw to jaw relation determined by condyles in the fossa.
- **Rest position** = determined largely by nm – activity and to a lesser degree by viscoelastic property of ms. Normal freeway space = 1 – 3 mm; the ms. are in minimum tonic-clonic contraction.
- **Bennett movement** = in lateral movement, the working-side condyle appears to rotate with a slight lateral shift in the direction of movement.
- Maximum opening = 50 – 60 mm
- Maximum lateral movement = 10 – 12 mm
- Maximum protrusive = 8 – 11 mm
- Maximum retrusion = 1 – 3 mm.

MUSCLES

- Superior head of lateral pterygoid M = active during jaw – closing movements only; as chewing and clenching; it stabilises the condylar head and disc against the articular eminence during closure.
- Inferior head = during jaw opening and protrusion only; assists in translation of condyle in D / F direction and contralaterally.
- Temporalis = is the principle positioner of mandible during elevation.
- DGA = by mylohyoid br of 5th N (Digastric posterior).
- DGP = by DG br of 7th N (Digastric posterior).
- Geniohyoid = by C1, C2 nerves.
- Tensor tympani and palati ms = by 5th n; control the auditory tube opening.

OCCLUSION

- By the **age of 9 mos**. = the width of arch has been established for both deciduous and permanent dentitions.
- Attrition of deciduous teeth = allows the mandibular to assume a more forward position during the growth period.
- Mandibular teeth erupt earlier than maxillary;
- Teeth in females are approx 5 mos earlier to males
- Arch perimeter in mandibular decreases by = 4 mm (Moorrees, 1959)
- Lower incisors erupt with approx 1.6 mm crowding is normal feature, it is a self-correcting anomaly.
- Normal maxillary and mandibular 6 relation is = ML cusp of maxillary 6 is in central fossa of mandibular 6; and MB cusp of maxillary 6 is in MB groove of mandibular 6.

DENTAL ARCH FORM

- Shape of arch form of facial surface of teeth = is a segment of ellipse.

- Arch form as defined by centroids = is a parabolic curve
- Mandibular arch curvature = is concave
- Maxillary arch curvature = is convex.
- Arch dimensions of maxillary > mandibular arch = so overjet is there and soft tissues are not caught b/w the teeth.

COMPENSATORY CURVES OF THE ARCHES

- Mandibular = concave
- Maxillary = convex
- **Bonwill** = U/L arches adapt themselves to a part of an equilateral triangle of 4" side, extending from a point b/w lower C.I to the condyle on both sides.
- **Curve of Spee** = within the AP / sagittal plane only; the cusps and incisal edges are arranged in a curved fashion. Depth measured in the mandibular premolar region.
- **Curve of Monson** = in the vertical plane; mandibular arch adapted itself to a curved segment of a sphere of 4" radius.
- **Thielmann's formula** of balanced occlusion in Complete dentures; aka **Hanau's quints** is = balance = CG . IG / CS. CH. PO.
- No posterior contacts during protrusive movements should be there.
- The IG should be increased in proportion to the severity of COS. The CH and PO remain the same.

ANGULATIONS

- Prolongation of axis lines bisecting the mandibular 7,8 tend to bisect lingual roots of maxillary 7,8 ; but of mandibular 6 when prolonged, passes b/w the buccal and lingual roots of maxillary 6.
- Supporting cusps = lingual in maxilla; buccal in mandible.
- **Center stops**, i.e. areas of contact in which supporting cusps rests are =

a. Central fossa of mandibular 6 = where ML cusp of maxillary 6 rests.

b. Central fossa of maxillary 6 = where DB cusp of mandibular 6 rests.

c. MB cusp of maxillary 6 = in MB groove of mandibular 6

d. Triangular ridge of MB cusp of maxillary 6 is slightly distal to the MB groove of mandibular 6.

e. DL cusps of mandibular molars = oppose the lingual sulcus of the lingual developmental groove.

CUSP AND FOSSA RELATIONSHIP

- DL cusps of maxillary molars = in the distal triangular fossa and marginal ridge of same mandibular molars and to the MMR of the distal molar tooth.
- Lingual cusps of maxillary 4,5 = in triangular fossa of mandibular 4,5.
- MB cusp of mandibular molars = in distal fossa or marginal ridge of the maxillary tooth mesial to its name sake tooth, i.e. mandibular 6 to the distal of maxillary 5.
- DB cusp of mandibular molar = in central fossa of maxillary molars.
- Buccal cusp tips of mandibular 5 = in mesial occlusal fossa of maxillary 5.
- Mandibular 4 = partly with maxillary 4 and maxillary 3.
- ML cusp of maxillary first molar = in central fossa of mand. 6.

RIDGE AND SULCUS APPOSITION

- Triangular ridge of buccal cusps of maxillary molars = in buccal grooves with their sulci in mandibular molars.
- Triangular ridge of DL cusp of mandibular 6 = in lingual groove and sulcus of maxillary 6.
- Oblique ridge of maxillary 6 (from DB to ML cusp) = fits in the sulcus formed on occlusal surface of mandibular 6 marked by the junction of DB, central and lingual develop grooves.

- There are **138 points** of occlusal contact in 32 teeth.
- **Group function** = multiple working side contacts.
- **Canine guided** = no contact on PM / M areas.

LATERAL OCCLUSAL RELATION OF TEETH

- During sliding contact action = the teeth intercuspate and slide over each other in a directional line **approx parallel with the oblique ridge of maxillary 6.** Oblique ridge of maxillary 6 is i.r.t. combined sulci of DB and occlusal develop grooves of mandibular 6.
- Cusp tip of mandibular 3 = through linguo-incisal embreasure b/w maxillary 2,3. Its distal cusp ridge contacts the mesial cusp ridge of maxillary 3.
- Cusp tip of mandibular 4 = through the occlusal embreasure of maxillary 3,4. Its MB ridge contacts distal cusp ridge of maxillary 3 and DB cusp ridge contacts MO slope of buccal cusp of maxillary 4.
- Lingual cusps of all premolars are out of contact until CR is attained. Then the only lingual cusps in contact are those of maxillary PM.
- The **tactile sensibility** in which the threshold values detecting foreign bodies b/w the teeth may be as little as **8 microns.**
- P.O. protective reflexes is due to **receptors** in PDL, TMJ etc.
- **Mesial migration** is due to = traction of **trans-septal fibres;** forces of mastication.
- Teeth and joint provide **passive guidance**; reflexes originating in receptors around the teeth give **active guidance**.

DEFINITIONS

Diphyodont	Man consists of 2 sets of dentitions, i.e. pri and permanent
Acrodont	Tooth is attached to crest of the bone; these are usually not replaced.
Anisognathus	Unequal jaws

DEFINITIONS (*Contd.*)

Ankylosis	Tooth attached to socket by bone
Bilophodont	The dentition in which there are fixed no. of cheek teeth at a time and are replaced by horizontal succession.
Bunodont	Conical cusps of tooth in primates.
Gomphosis	Tooth is attached to socket by PDL.
Haplodont / reptilian	**Simplest form of teeth,** with conical form of crown and root; single cone.
Heterodont	Human consist of different sets of teeth, i.e. incisors, C, PM; M.
Isognathus	Having equal jaws.
Monophyodont	Which consist of only one set of the teeth.
Pleurodont	Tooth is attached to inner margin of bone. These can be replaced.
Thecodont	PD membrane do not undergo significant changes.

No. of developmental lobes in teeth

- Primary incisor 1
- Permanent incisor 4
- Permanent canine 4
- Premolars 4
- 3 – cusped lower PM 5
- max E 5
- max 6 5
- mand E 5
- all other permanent molars 4

Root morphology

- Anterior tooth which is least likely to variation in root morphology = max 3
- Anterior teeth likely to have bifurcated RC = mand 3 = facial and lingual
- Premolar with 2 roots and 2 RC = max 4
- Teeth with round blunt roots easy for extraction = max 1 and mand 5
- Teeth with roots that are thin MD, wider BL and mesial and distal concavities = mand 1; DB root of max 6; roots of mand molars;
- Two RC = in mand 3 and mesial root of mand 6.
- Largest root which shows facial and lingual concavities = palatal root of max 6
- Teeth show great variations in root morphology = third molars
- longest root = max 3
- Max molar having *trifurcation* of root as mesial = 3 mm, closest to the CEJ; buccal is 4 mm; distal is 5 mm (ie M,B,D = 3,4,5)
- Roots of mand molars are oriented in = DB direction
- Size of roots of max. 6 = P>MB>DB root

CONTACT AREAS

TEETH	MAXILLARY		MANDIBULAR	
	Mesial	**Distal**	**Mesial**	**Distal**
1	Incisal 3rd	Jn. of Incisal and mid 3rd	Incisal 3rd	Incisal 3rd
2	Jn. of Incisal and mid 3rd	mid 3rd	Incisal 3rd	Incisal 3rd
3	Jn. of Incisal and mid 3rd	mid 3rd	Incisal 3rd	Jn. of Incisal and mid 3rd

CONTACT AREAS

TEETH	MAXILLARY		MANDIBULAR	
	Mesial	**Distal**	**Mesial**	**Distal**
4	Jn. of occlusal and mid 3rd	Jn. of occlusal and mid 3rd	Jn. of occlusal and mid 3rd	Jn. of occlusal and mid 3rd
5	Jn. of occlusal and mid 3rd	Jn. of occlusal and mid 3rd	Jn. of occlusal and mid 3rd	Jn. of occlusal and mid 3rd
6	Jn. of occlusal and mid 3rd	Jn. of occlusal and mid 3rd	Jn. of occlusal and mid 3rd	Jn. of occlusal and mid 3rd
7	Jn. of occlusal and mid 3rd	mid 3rd	Jn. of occlusal and mid 3rd	mid 3rd

- contact areas b/w posterior teeth are located facially and occlusally from the center of the proximal surface.

Table of age and crown completion stage

Age	**Permanent Crown completed**
2 ½–3 yrs	First molars
4–5 yrs	Central and lateral incisors
5–6 yrs	First PM
6–7	Canine; 2nd PM
7–8 yrs	2nd molars
12–16 yrs	3rd molars

- A tooth erupts in the oral cavity after approx 4 yrs of its crown completion.
- Root completion / apical end closure of a tooth occurs approx 3 yrs after the eruption.

Teeth	No. of cusps	No. of pulp horns	No. of dev. Lobes
Deci A	——	2; mesial and distal	1
B	—-	2; mesial and distal	1
C	1	1	4
D	4	4	4
E	5	5	5
Permanent 1,2	—	♦ 3 = max 1 ♦ 2 = max 2 ♦ 2 = mand 1,2	4
3	1	1	4
4,5 and mand 4	2	2	4
Mand 5	3	3	5
6	5	Max = 3 Mand = 4	5
7	4	max = 3 mand = 4	4
8	Max = 3 Mand = 4; variable	Max = 3 Mand = 4	4

Teeth	Occlusal outline	Cervical outline
Max 4	Hexagonal	Kidney-shaped
Max 5	Oval / more rounded	Oval
Max 6	Rhomboidal	Rhomboidal
Max 7	Rhomboidal	Rhomboidal
Max 8	Heart shaped	Variable

Teeth	Occlusal outline	Cervical outline
Mand 4	Roughly diamond-shaped	Variable
Mand 5	Square = if 3 cusped Round = if 2 cusped	Variable
Mand 6	Trapezoid or rectangular	Quadrilateral
Mand 7	Rectangular	Quadrilateral

EMBREASURE

Max teeth	Labial	Lingual
1,1	V shape	Wider
1,2	V shape	Wider
2,3	Emb. changed due to a **definite convexity at mesio-labial line** angle of canine	
3,4		A **concavity in DL line angle** of 3 and a developmental groove crossing MMR of 1st PM.
4,5		
5,6		**ML lobe of 6 is larger so** the embr is smaller.
6,7 / 7,8		ML and DL line angles are rounded and **so lingual embr are open.**

Embreasure in mand teeth

Mand teeth	Labial	Lingual
2,3	Influenced by prominent mesiolabial line angle of 3	

Embreasure in mand teeth (*Contd.*)

Mand teeth	Labial	Lingual
3,4		Opened up due to a *slight concavity* on 3 DL and a ML dev groove across MR of 4.
4,5	Distal surface of 4 describes **a larger arc;** mesial surface of 5 is broad	Wide due to the **lingual convergence of 4** and narrow lingual cusp forms
5,6	Mesial contact area of 6 is BUCCAL than on any other mand posterior teeth ; **mesial outline tapers to lingual** and forms a generous lingual embr.	
6,7 ; 7,8	Distal CA of 6 is not broad; rounded DB line angle; embr. wider than at mesial of 6	embr. wider than at mesial of 6

PULP CAVITIES

Max 1 = triangular

Max 2 = triangular

Max 3 = ellipitical; **largest pulp chamber buccolingually**

Max 4 = **kidney shaped**; due to a mesial developmental groove

Max 5 = **oval**

Max 6 = rhomboidal in shape with rounded corners

Max 7 = MB line angle is more acute and DB angle is more obtuse than ML.

Mand 1 and 2 = round / oval

Mand 3 = oval / triangular

(dentinal islands found in any tooth that demonstrates an extremely wide labiolingual dim and a narrow MD dim.; found in mand 3 and max 5.)

Mand 4 , 5 = oval / triangular/ rectangular

Mand 6 = quadrilateral

Mand 7 = triangular

Mand 8 = rectangular / triangular

Miscellaneous points and important features

- Max 2 likely to have a lingual groove that extends from the enamel onto the cemental area of the root.
- Max 2 has a lingual pit.
- Roots of max 3 is LONGEST;
- Longest crown is of = mand 3
- The apex of permanent tooth closes after = 2 – 3 yrs of eruption.
- Root development of permanent dentition except 3rd molars is completed by 16 yrs; crown up to 8 yrs.
- Primary molars differ from permanent molars in that pri molars have flatter facial and lingual surfaces from occlusal to cervical ridges.
- Maxillary D has an occlusal surface that most often bears the greatest resemblance to premolar.
- Anatomic feature that is **most likely to complicate root planning** of a max 2 = is distolingual groove.
- Max 4 have sharp demarcations b/w pulp chambers and pulp canals.
- Mand 4 has only one pulp horn or it may have 2 pulp horns.
- Calcification of mand 8 begins at 8 – 10 yrs age.
- Maxillary tooth crown exhibits **concavities mesial** of first PM and distal of max first molars.
- In ideal intercuspal relation in a normal dentition, each of tooth contact 2 teeth except max 8 and mand 1.

- **Size of pulp horns** from largest to smallest is:
- Max 6 = MB > M L > DB > DL
- Mand 6 = MB > ML > DB > DL > D
- **Size of cusps** =
- Max 6 = ML > MB > DB > D L
- Mand 6 = MB > ML > DL > DB > D
- Size of cusps in mand 5 = buccal > ML > DL
- In cervical cross section, the root of a mand canine is described as flattened in mesiodistal direction.
- The largest incisal / occlusal embreasure is located b/w the max 2 and 3.
- At birth, on r/g, 24 teeth are present.
- First evidence of calcification at birth is of first molars.
- Last primary tooth to be replaced by permanent tooth = max C
- Permanent 7, 8 and premolars buds are = initiated after birth.
- DL is the deepest groove on occlusal surface of max 6.
- Mand 4 is smallest among all the premolars.
- Max 6 has the largest root trunk.
- A mand 5 is tilted lingually so the gingival sulcus is most affected lingually.
- Average maxillary arch length = 128 mm.
- Total occlusal contact points in dentition = 138
- No. of centric stops in maxillary arch = 7
- **No. of centric stops in mandibular arch** = 6
- Average virtual length a mandible moves in a chewing cycle is = 16 – 20 mm.
- Buccal surface of mand posterior teeth are mesial to outer surface of ramus.
- Midline foramina of incisive canal is ka **foramen of Scarpa**.
- The tip of mand 3 during lateral working movement passes through mesial to the tip of max 3.

- In centric occlusion, lingual cusp of mand 4 contacts with no other tooth in any arch.
- When a protrusive mand movement is done, i.e. anterior teeth edge to edge, the mand 6 has a potential to contact 5 and 6.
- In an acquired class III cross bite relation, as the mandible retrudes the max 2 contacts canines and lateral incisors.
- The palatal root tip of max 6 is likely to be forced into the maxillary sinus during surgical removal, b'coz it is the longest root.
- Styloglossus = is extrinsic ms of tongue; functions to retract the tongue.
- Translation is condylar movement performed as the mandible moves from a pure protrusive movement from maximum intercuspal position to maximum protruded position.
- Mand lateral translation / Bennett movement occurs during the earliest stage of lateral movement; occurs on working side; condyle moves downward—forward—mesially.
- Protrusive movement is produced by contraction of the lateral pterygoid m.
- Mand 4 has non- functional lingual cusps.
- Max 4 is the most difficult tooth for RCT.
- As the mouth is opened widely, the articular disc moves anteriorly i.r.t. articular eminence.
- The **first succedaneous tooth** to erupt = mand 1
- **Last succedaneous tooth** to erupt = max 3
- Upper lateral is the last incisor to erupt.
- **Mamelons are absent in primary dentitions**.
- Mand D has a prominent transverse ridge on its occlusal table.
- An **outstanding feature of mand D** = typically curved cervical line on buccal surface. Distal part of crown is shorter than mesial part, so **cervical line** DIPS APICALLY where it joins the mesial root.
- Max D has most resemblance to PMs.
- Mand D has most unique buccal cervical bulge or ridge.

- Mand D has a prominent transverse ridge.
- Mand D and max D resemble nothing in permanent dentition completely.
- Mand E and max E resemble mand 6 and max 6 respectively.

Organ	Tissue formed	Origin
Enamel organ	Enamel	Ectodermal
Dental papillae	Dentin and pulp	Mesenchymal
Dental sac	Cementum and PDL	Mesenchymal

Principal fibres	Periodontal fibres
They **do not attach** to the alveolar bone	They **attach to the alveolar bone**
Dentogingival	Alveolar crest fibres
Dentoperiosteal	Horizontal
Trans-septal	Oblique ; **maximum in no.**
Circular	Apical

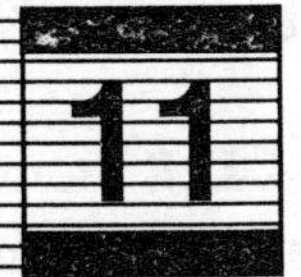

Dental Histology

DEVELOPMENT AND GROWTH OF TEETH

Ist enamel organs to appear = are of mandibular anterior region.

IEE, OEE, SR, Stratum intermedium develop in this sequence.

Enamel organ: Ectodermal origin. Main function of epithelial cells is to **form (Enamel) - enamel organ**

Dental papilla: Formed from ectomesenchymal cells, Cells of **dental papilla** -form **Pulp and dentin.**

Dental sac: Formed from ectomesenchymal cells and fibres surrounding enamel organ + Dental papilla, Cells of **dental sac** –form **Cementum and PDL.**

Tooth formation is similar to exocrine gland because a proliferation of basal cells occurs.

Stellate reticulum appears in cap stage, known as enamel pulp. **Stellate reticulum** collapses before enamel formation begins.

Enamel knot and enamel cord disappear before enamel formation begins—Act as RESERVOIR of dividing cells for growing enamel organs.

IEE - form Ameloblasts (40 μ height × 4–5 μ width).

Has an organizing influence on mesenchyme of dental papilla to form ODONTOBLASTS before enamel formation starts.

Membrana performativa—is basement membrane which separates enamel organ and dental papilla before the dentin formation.

Hertwig sheath initiates radicular dentin formation, has **only OEE and IEE.**

> With the formation of dentin —the cells of IEE differentiate into ameloblasts → to deposit enamel.
>
> **Enamel does not form in absences of dentin**
>
> so dentin formation precedes and is essential for enamel formation.

Advanced bell stage - Outlines future DEJ.

> ⇒ Bone = Type I collagen (93%)
>
> ⇒ PDL = collagen (type I) fibers
>
> ⇒ In dentinogenesis imperfecta = type III collagen
>
> ⇒ Basement membrane = type IV collagen

Structure first formed by tooth bud which remains in evidence in the formed tooth is = DEJ.

ENAMEL

⇒ Thickness on cusps of M/PM = 2–2.5 mm (maximum)

⇒ Thickness at neck of tooth = knife-edge

⇒ Hardest calcified tissue of the body; brittle

⇒ Dentin is abraded 15–25 times more than enamel.

⇒ Cementum is abraded 35 times more than enamel.

Chemical properties

> ⇒ Enamel matrix mineralisation begins immediately after it is secreted.
>
> ⇒ The LAG in mineralisation after matrix formation is greater in dentin than in bone.

⇒ **Hypocalcified structure** in enamel = Tufts, lamellae, Retzius lines.

⇒ **Last organic matrix** secreted by ameloblasts = Primary cuticle.

⇒ **Layer of cells which is essential to enamel formation but does not actually secrete the enamel is stratum intermedium.**

STRIATIONS: Transverse striations demarcate rod segments, more pronounced in enamel which is insufficiently calcified. Rods are segmented because enamel is formed in a rhythmic manner.

⇒ Rods are approx. more parallel to long axis in body/head and deviate about 65° from long axis, as they fan out in tails.

<u>Direction of rods</u>

⇒ Cervical and central parts of crown of <u>primary tooth</u> = approx. HORIZONTAL

⇒ Nearing the incisal edge / cusp tip = OBLIQUE

⇒ Edge / tip of cusp= VERTICAL

⇒ Cervical area of <u>permanent teeth</u> = APICAL DIRECTION

GNARLED ENAMEL

Bundles of rods seem to interwine more irregularly, found near the dentin **in the area of cusps or incisal edges.**

HUNTER-SCHREGER BANDS: regular change in the direction of rods is the functional adaptation. **Origin at DEJ** and pass out ending at some distance from outer enamel surface.

Increment lines of Retzius (like growth rings of tree), i.e. successive apposition of layers of enamel during crown formation.

Surfaces structures of enamel

1. **Structureless layer** = 30 μm thick, in 70% of permanent teeth and all deciduous teeth.

   ⇒ More <u>heavily mineralised than the bulk of enamel</u> beneath it.

HS bands	Origin at DEJ	Due to different organic contents, rod directions	Resist risk of cleavage along axial direction
Enamel lamella	Origin at enamel surface	Hypomineralised	along plane of tension
Enamel tufts	Origin at DEJ	Hypomineralised	
Enamel cracks	Origin at DEJ, perpendicular to DEJ		
Lines of Retzius		Variation in structure and mineralisation	
Structureless layer		Hypermineralised	

2. **Perikymata**

⇒ Believed to be the external manifestations of striae of Retzius.

3. **Cracks**

⇒ Are the outer edges of lamellae, originate at DEJ.

4. **Neonatal line**

⇒ Marked by accentuated lines of Retzius.

⇒ Prenatal enamel is better developed, because it is formed in a protected intrauterine environment.

5. **Primary enamel cuticle**

⇒ Known as Nasmyth's membrane.

⇒ Secreted by Ameloblasts **after enamel formation is complete**.

6. **Enamel lamellae (hypomineralised)**

   By careful decalcification —lamella persist, cracks disappear.

7. **DEJ Scalloped line (pitted DEJ)**

   ⇒ Convexities of scallops toward dentin.

8. **Odontoblast processes and enamel spindles**

   ⇒ Odontoblast processes pass through DEJ into enamel, many are thickened at their end - known as E. spindles.

Age changes

⇒ Facial and lingual surfaces lose their structure much more rapidly than proximal surfaces.

⇒ Anterior teeth loss more rapidly than posterior teeth.

Development

⇒ Enamel organ is ectodermal.

⇒ **Cervical loop** – at the wide basal opening of enamel organ, IEE reflects onto the OEE, forms Hertwig's root sheath.

⇒ **stimulus which initiates actual formation of enamel matrix is-presence of predentin.**

⇒ Stage 1: Shape of DEJ and crown is determined.

⇒ Stage 2: Reversal of polarity of cells of IEE and nutritional source

⇒ Stage 3: PO dentin is necessary for beginning of enamel formation.

⇒ Stage 5: After complete maturation of enamel, the ameloblasts change to – REE which protects enamel by separating it from CT until tooth erupts.

Tome's processes: are projections of ameloblasts in enamel matrix.

⇒ **Tome's process show Picket-Fence arrangement.**

⇒ Rods are at an angle to ameloblasts and Tome's process.

⇒ 4-Ameloblasts (hexagonal) are involved to form a ROD (Keyhole-shape rod).

First mineral is in the form of crystalline apatite. Maturation of enamel is = increase in % of inorganic content and decrease in organic and water content.

Maturation of bone = increase in % of inorganic content and decrease in water content, and little change in organic and collagen contents.

⇒ Maturation starts from Height of crown and progresses cervically

⇒ Begins at dentinal end of rods. So, integration of 2 processes.

⇒ **Loss in volume of organic matrix is due to withdrawal of protein and water.**

⇒ Surface layer of enamel is structureless and more radiopaque than enamel bulk below it (hypermineralised).

DENTIN

Predentin	Non calcified	First formed, adjacent to pulp; 2–6 μ wide
Primary dentin	Mentle dentin + Circumpulpal dentin	Formed before root completion
Secondary		Formed after root completion
Peritubular	Most calcified	Immediately surrounds the tubules
Interglobular	Hypocalcified	In crowns, just below mantle dentin, defect in mineralisation
Neonatal line	Hypocalcified	
Incremental line of **Von-Ebner**	Highly calcified	
Contour line of **Owen**	Hypocalcified	
Sclerotic or transparent	Hypercalcified	Refractive index equalised, esp. in roots, mineralised D. tubule; no odontoblastic process

DENTIN (*Contd.*)

Intertubular	Highly mineralised	Main body of dentin
Root dentin		Tome's granular layer
Mentle dentin (Primary)		First formed along cuspal tips in crown, **Korff's fibers**
Tome's granular layer	In root only	Adjacent to cementum **(root dentin)**; formed by terminal parts of dentinal tubules.
Dead tracts		Degenerated odontoblast process
Terminal bar apparatus of odontoblasts		Is near pulp – predentin border and is without organellos
Circumpulpal (Primary)	more mineralised than mantle	All dentin prior to root completion, forms remaining primary Dentin/bulk
Tertiary, reparative or response Dentin		

⇒ Difference between dentin and bone = osteocytes in bone, but only **odontoblast processes in dentin.**

⇒ Incremental lines of Retzius (enamel) = lines of Owen (in dentin).

⇒ **Mantle dentin = is first formed dentin.**

⇒ Structure **essential for initiation of dentin formation** = IEE

STRUCTURE

⇒ **Dentinal tubules** – are the odontoblastic processes, follow a gentle S curve in crown, less so in roots.

⇒ Ratio between outer : inner surface of dentin = 5:1

⇒ Diameter = 3–4 μm = near pulp (layer)
1–μm = at outer ends

⇒ No. of tubules/area = Pulpal: outer surface = 4:1

⇒ No. of tubules near pulpal end = 50000–90000/mm^2

⇒ Some tubules **cross DEJ** and enter enamel = as **ENAMEL SPINDLES.**

TUBULIN- protein present throughout dentin.

Mature dentin contains collagen, but enamel contains keratin.

Collagen contains hydroxyproline and hydrolysine residues.

PRIMARY DENTIN

a. **Mantle** = Ist formed dentin in crown underlying DEJ
b. **Circumpulpal dentin**: Forms remaining primary dentin/bulk of tooth

⇒ all dentin prior to root completion.

⇒ slightly more mineral than Mantle dentin.

SECONDARY DENTIN: after root completion.

⇒ Fewer tubules than primary dentin.

TERTIARY DENTIN: reparative/response dentin.

⇒ Formed as a proliferative response against any trauma, etc.

INCREMENTAL LINES **(Von Ebner)**

⇒ also known as Imbrication Lines, due to daily rhythm.

⇒ <u>**Contour lines (of Owen)**</u> – Some lines accentuated due to disturbances in matrix and mineralisation process – are HYPO-CALCIFIED BANDS.

⇒ **NEONATAL Line – Hypocalcified**

INTERGLOBULAR DENTIN

⇒ Hypomineralised area:

INNERVATION OF DENTIN

⇒ Nerve endings in predentin and inner dentin = upto 100–150 μm from the pulp, esp. in pulphorns.

Theories of pain transmission

⇒ Fluid /hydrodynamic theory - most popular.

Development - Dentinogenesis

⇒ Begins at cusp tips

⇒ Daily rate of formation – is **4 μm/day** of dentin till crown is formed, teeth erupt and come in occlusion, then dentiogenesis slows to 1 μ / day

⇒ But reparative dentin is formed 4 μ / day

⇒ **Korff's Fibres** – the initial dentin deposition <u>along the cusp tips.</u>

⇒ H/E = Root dentin is distinguished readily from crown dentin by presence of = **Tomes granular layer.**

PULP

⇒ Pulp starts developing at 8th week IU (in primary teeth)

⇒ Total vol. of permanent pulp = 0.38 cc

⇒ Mean vol. of single adult pulp = 0.02 cc

⇒ Molar pulps = 3–4 × the incisor pulp

⇒ Smallest pulp = lower central incisor = 0.006 cc

⇒ Largest pulp = upper first molar = 0.068 cc

⇒ Pulp of lower third molar is larger than upper third molar by (0.031 > 0.023 cc)

Apical foramen

⇒ Av. size in adults – (upper) = 0.4 mm

⇒ Av. size in adults – (lower) = 0.3 mm

⇒ Apical foramen of fully developed tooth is lined by cementum at CDJ/apical constriction area, i.e. a layer of cementum covers the dentin inside the RC upto apical constriction area.

Accessory canals = mainly maximum in **apical 3rd of root.**

Occur where sheath cells are lost prematurely (or) developing root encounters a blood vessel.

Structural features: 3 zones

⇒ **Odontoblast zone**

⇒ **Cell free (Weil's) zone** – in which odontoblasts move pulpward during tooth development.

⇒ **Cell rich zone** mainly fibroblast and undifferentiated messen-chymal cells.

FIBROBLASTS: pulp lacks elastic fibers.

⇒ **Most numerous cells** and form collagen.

Pulp organ

⇒ has no elastic fibres, **no parasympathetic and proprioceptive fibres,** has mainly fibroblasts,

⇒ **Histiocystes are macrophages of pulp.**

Odontoblasts: 2nd most prominent cells in pulp.

⇒ Lie adjacent to predentin (in odontogenic zone)

⇒ Area near the pulp – predentin junction is devoid of organelles. This **clear area** + adjacent intercellular junction is known as **terminal bar apparatus of odontoblasts.**

Blood vessels

⇒ Pulpal pressure is among the **highest** of the body tissue.

⇒ Blood flow in arterioles = 0.3–1.0 mm/sec
in venules = 0.15 mm/sec
in capillaries = 0.08 mm/sec

NERVES

⇒ **No parasymp. fibres = so only pain sensation is felt.**

⇒ Principal type of nerves in pulp are = Symp. and afferent fibres, i.e. **A-delta and C fibres.** (Also refer section on endodontics.)

⇒ Sympathetic in nature = vasoconstriction

A-delta carry shoup, localised pain—First pain. (@ 100 m/sec.)

C fibres carry throbbing pain/slow—second pain. (@ 0.5–2 m/sec.)

⇒ Larger fibres = 5–13 μm

⇒ Majority of fibres = < 4 μm

⇒ Large myelinated fibres = A-delta;

⇒ Small unmyelinated fibres = C-fibres

Plexue of Rashkow: lies adjacent to cell rich zone.

Nerve terminals

⇒ Mainly **sensory recepters.**

⇒ are non-myelinated but enclosed in Schwann cell covering.

⇒ Sensory response in pulp **can not differentiate** between heat, touch, pressure, chemicals, but **only pain** to all stimuli - because pulp lack specific receptors.

Function

⇒ **First /primary role of pulp anlage-induction of oral epithelium differentiation into dental lamina and enamel organ formation.**

⇒ also induces the developing enamel organ to become particular type of tooth.

Pulp stones or denticles

1. **True denticles**: Structure same as dentin, i.e. have dentinal tubuli and odontoblast processes.
2. **False denticles**: Seen as concentric layers of calcified tissues, no dentinal tubules.
3. **Diffuse calcification**: Usually present in root canals and less often in coronal area, whereas denticles (1, 2) are seen frequently in coronal pulp.

Free denticles: Entirely surrounded by pulp tissues.

Attached denticles: Partly fused with dentin.

Embedded denticles: Entirely surrounded by dentin.

DEVELOPMENT

⇒ Dental papilla is known as pulp only after dentin forms around it, dental papilla controls early tooth formation and shape of tooth.

⇒ **Odland body** are keratinosomes (lamellar granules)

CEMENTUM

⇒ Avascular

⇒ It has **highest F^- content** of all the mineralised tissues, has type – I collagen.

⇒ *Cementogenesis*: It is preceded by dentin deposition along the inner aspect of Hertwig's root sheath, which then breaks and CT contact dentin–so **Undifferentiated Mesenchymal Cells** from CT form cementocytes to form cementum.

⇒ Fenestration of Hertwig's epithelium root sheath is very necessary for cementum to be deposited during root development.

⇒ **Cementoid = uncalcified matrix**

⇒ Embedded part of CT PDL fibres in cementum = **Sharpey's** fibres

⇒ **Acellular** - from CEJ to apex, but often **missing on apical 3rd** root (where only **cellular cementum**) exists

⇒ Acellular cementum = on coronal half of root

⇒ Cellular cementum = on apical half of root

⇒ Thinnest at CEJ = 20–50 μ

⇒ **Thickest towards apex = 150–200** μ

⇒ Attachment proper of Sharpey's fibers is confined to most superficial or recently formed cementum.

⇒ Peripheral portion of Sharpey's fibers are more mineralised than central parts.

INCREMENTAL LINES are highly mineralised areas, with less collagen and more ground substance.

Cemento-dentinal junction

⇒ smooth = in permanent teeth

⇒ scalloped = in deci. Teeth

⇒ Sometimes, intermediate cementum layer exists between cementum and dentin, predominantly in apical 2/3rds of roots of M and PMs and rarely on incisors and primary teeth (also known as Hyaline layer of Hopewell and Smith).

CEJ

⇒ 30% = sharp line junction

⇒ 10% = C and E do not meet

⇒ 60% = cementum overlaps enamel for a short distance.

FUNCTIONS

⇒ **Primary function** = to furnish a <u>medium for attachment</u> of collagen fibers which bind the tooth with alveolar bone

<u>Anatomic repair</u>

⇒ former outline of root surface is re-established by cementum formation

<u>Functional repair</u>

⇒ only a thin layer of cementum is formed, rest of PDL space is restored by bone-growth in the area of resorption.

PERIODONTAL LIGAMENT

⇒ also known as <u>Desmodont; gomphosis</u>

⇒ PDL formation occurs after the cells of Hertwig's sheath have separated forming rests of Malassez

⇒ Osteoclasts: formed by fusion of monocytes.

⇒ Progenitor cells - located predominantly near the blood vessels

Fibers

⇒ majority of fibres = collagen

⇒ Elastic fibers = only in walls of blood vessels.

Collagen: esp. **type I collagen** in PDL - contain hydroxyproline and some type III also. Most numerous, constitute main attachment of the tooth.

Nerve fibers

⇒ large dia/myelinated, concerned with touch.

⇒ **Small dia. fibers = with pain.**

Primary role = support

⇒ Collagen of PDL turnover is **fastest** of all CT of body.

CLINICAL CONSIDERATION

⇒ PDL width ranges from 0.15 mm to 0.38 mm

⇒ Thinnest in middle region of root, as there is **fulcrum of physiologic movement**, hourglass shaped.

Cortical plates

⇒ thickest in PM and M regions of L jaw, esp. on buccal side.

⇒ Alveolar crest's shape depends on position of teeth. Inclination of tooth is most pronounced in PM and M region esp. mesially and so alv. crest is slopes distally.

⇒ **Canals of ZuckerKandl and Hirschfield** (Nutrient canals) are in I/dental and inter radicular septa, which house A, V, N and lymph vessels.

⇒ Osteoblasts secretes **type I collagen** and non-collagenous matrix, i.e. osteoid (mineralization lags behind the bone matrix production)

ORAL MUCOUS MEMBRANE

⇒ 3 types:

1. Masticatory - gingiva, hard palate
   bound to bone and does not stretch
2. Lining / reflecting - lip, cheek, vestibular fornix

(All surfaces except dorsum of tongue and masticatory mucosa)

- Alv. mucosa, floor of mouth
- soft palate
- distensible and adopting to ms/jaw movements.

3. Specialised (Sensory) mucosa - Dorsum of tongue, Taste buds

Basement membrane =

⇒ fine (reticulin) fibers

⇒ in skin = it has leminin and fibronectin, type IV collagen, etc.

Submucosa

⇒ Here only, larger As divide into smaller branches.

⇒ nerve fibers in submucosa are **myelinated**.

EPITHELIUM

⇒ **Keratinised** - gingiva and hard palate

⇒ **Non-keratinised** - cheek, faucial, sublingual tissues.

⇒ All epithelium cells contain keratin intermediate filaments (7–11 nm wide)

⇒ CT cells have vimentin filaments.

⇒ ms. cells have desmin filaments

⇒ Ns cells have neural filaments.

4- layers, i.e. BSGC (in skin, there are BSGLC)

⇒ Str. basal

⇒ Str. spinosum (Prickle cell layer)

⇒ Str. granulosum

⇒ Str. cornium

⇒ Basal layers and parabasal spinous layer are known as **Str. germinativum** (as mitosis occurs there)

⇒ Basal lamina–two parts

1. Lamina lucida = just below epith. Cells, contains laminin and Bullous pemphigoid antigen.
2. Lamina Densa - Adjacent to CT, has **type IV collagen**
   - Antigen bound by **antibody KF-1**

⇒ Of the 4 layers, the **spinous cells are the most active in protein synthesis.**

⇒ **Str. granulosum** - cells contain **keratohyalin** granules.

⇒ **Odland body** (also known as keratinosome) is an organelle in upper spinous and granular cells layers

NON-KER. EPITHELIUM- 3 layers

⇒ Str. basale

⇒ Str. intermedium

⇒ Str. superficiale

⇒ **No str. granulosum**

HARD PALATE

⇒ Anterolateral (fatty) zone

⇒ Posterolateral (glandular) zone

Difference between submucosa of HP and gingiva.

A distinct submucosa can't be recognised in gingiva.

⇒ Most outstanding difference between gingiva and mucosa of hard palate is = PO glands

⇒ In hard palate and gingiva = lamina propria is directly attached to bone, without an intervening submucosa.

Jacobson's organs - is vomeronasal organ;

Lined by olfactory epithelium, is seen in 12–15 week IU, after which it undergoes involution.

Gingiva - extends from DG junction to alv. mucosa,

⇒ Dense lamina propria, lacks a separate submucosa

⇒ Mucogingival junction separates the gingiva from alv. mucosa.

⇒ Stippling: portions of epithelium are elevated and in between elevation - there are depressions (which are the center of heavier epithelium, ridges)

⇒ **Stippling is absent in infants**.

⇒ Stippling is due to heavier epithelial ridges, causing depressed center.

I/D papilla

⇒ triangular from buccal view
⇒ tent / shape—posterior teeth
⇒ pyramidal—anterior teeth

Col- depressed part of (tent) gingiva, which fits below the contact area.

⇒ non-keratinised epithelium. and so more vulnerable to PD diseases.

Diff. between gingiva and alv. mucosa?

⇒ gingiva is immovably attached to periosteum of alv. bone, but submucosa of alv. mucosa is loosely textured,

Merkel cells - are specialised neural, pressure-sensitive, receptor cells.

Specialised mucosa

(also refer section on orthodontics)

⇒ **Filiform papilla — No taste buds** (maximum, velvetty appearance)
⇒ Fungiform - 1–3 taste buds
⇒ Vallate - 8-10, numerous taste buds, have Von-Ebner glands opening which are main source of salivary lipase.
⇒ Foliate - have taste buds

Dev. of JE

⇒ **Primary enamel cuticle** (PEC) is formed by ameloblasts after completion of enamel matrix.

⇒ **REE** ameloblasts decrease in size, and enamel organ is decreased to a few layers of flat cuboidal cells.

⇒ Remnants of PEC after eruption = known as **nasmyth's membrane.**

⇒ Once the tip of tooth has erupted = REE is known as **primary attachment epithelium (PAE)**

SALIVARY GLANDS

⇒ Most mportant function = saliva production and secretion

⇒ SGs ›resent everywhere in oral cavity, except a portion of anterior part of hard palate

Mucous cells

⇒ Its secretory products differ from serous products.

⇒ Ratio of carbohydrate to protein is greater

⇒ Large amounts of sialic acid and sulfated sugar residues present.

Parotid and Von- Ebner's	- **serous**
Sublingual	- mucous (predominantly mucous)
Submandibular	- mixed, predominantly serous
Glands of Blandin and Nuhn	- mucous

⇒ **Lingual** – in groups as :

Anterior lingual glands known as glands of Blandin and Nuhn.

Posterior lingual glands known as Von Ebner's glands. Purely serous, ducts open in trough of vallate papilla and at foliate papilla.

⇒ **Mixed gland** - esp. mucous

DUCTS

1. Within a lobule, the smallest ducts are ; **intercalated ducts** (low cuboid cells)
2. Connect to **striated duct** (tall, columnar cells)
3. Main excretory duct **interlobular ducts** (pseudostratified cells)

⇒ **Final saliva = Hypotonic,**
⇒ Maximum saliva = from SMG (60%)
⇒ Primary saliva obtained from intercalated duct is - Isotonic or slightly hypertonic to plasma.
⇒ Secretion obtained from excretory duct is hypotonic.

1. **Watery saliva = p.symp. stimulation**, Copious quantity
2. **Thicker**: less quantity of saliva : by **symp stimulation**

Parotid and Von- Ebner's	- Stensen's duct
Sublingual	- Bartholin's duct
Submandibular	- Wharton's duct

SALIVA: composition (physiology)

⇒ 750 ml/day = 60% by SMG
30% by parotid
15% by SLG
7% by minor SG

⇒ $H2O$ = 99%
⇒ pH = 6.7–7.4
⇒ pH of parotid saliva = 6.0 – 7.8
⇒ Primary buffering system of saliva = HCO_3
⇒ Main category of org. subs. in saliva = Secretory proteins, esp. for $Ca–PO_4$ hemostasin and pellicle formation.

Immunoglobulins

⇒ Main is = Ig A (Salivary IgA)

⇒ It differs from serum IgA by;

- produced locally by plasma cells
- has dimer of two IgA molecules
  + and a protein known as J-chain
  + secretory component - which facilitates transfer of IgA to the lumen.

Ig acts primarily by inhibiting the adherence of bacteria to oral tissues.

Lactoferrin: It enhances inhibitory effect of Ab on the bacteria.

ERUPTION

(See section on orthodontics)

⇒ Upper permanent molars, develop in tuberosity, have their occlusal surfaces facing distally.

⇒ Lower permanent molars develop with occ. surfaces mesially and become upright when space becomes available.

⇒ Successional teeth possess gubernacular canal and G. cord - filled CT and epithelium ramnant of D. lamina - helps in guiding permanent tooth during eruption.

⇒ **Cushion-hammock ligament** acts as sling and base, against which the growing root gets an occlusal thrust for eruption.

⇒ Trans septal lig. has a key role in maintaining tooth position and in mesial drift.

Root stumps

⇒ mostly in realation to premolars esp.mand. second, because mostly roots of primary mand second molars are strongly curved and divergent.

Retained primary teeth

Mostly max lateral incisors Less frequently primary Mand second molars Least frequently mand central incisors If permanent ankylosed – then primary retained, e.g. mostly primary and secondary canines.

TMJ DEVELOPMENT

⇒ At approx. 10 weeks, components appear.

⇒ At approx. 12 week, articular disc and 2 joint cavities appear.

⇒ Pain in TMJ is transmitted by the auriculotemporal N in the capsule and periphery of the disk.

⇒ Large central area of Disc = **avascular** and without nerves, has limited reparative ability.

⇒ Normal interincisal dis = 48 mm – male

⇒ = 45.5 mm – female

⇒ Mandibular deviates mostly to **left**

⇒ In MPDS ms tenderness – mostly Lateral pterygoid, > temporalis > Mesial pterygoid > masseter.

Special points

1. No. of rods in enamel = 5 millions in mand lateral incisors. to 12 millions in maxillary first molars.
2. Structureless layer of enamel = 30 microns thick
3. Size of ameloblast = 40 micron (h) × 4–5 microns dia.
4. Size of ameloblast body = 40 × 7 microns
5. Size/ dia of ameloblast process = 3–4 micron at pulpal end, 1 micron at DEJ.
6. Width of PDL = 0.15–0.38 mm
7. Size of enamel prism/rod = 9 × 5 × 4 micron (l, b, d).
8. Diameter of enamel rods at outer end : dentinal end = 2 : 1
9. Enamel crystals = 8 times thicker than dentin.

10. Size of hydroxyapatite crystals of enamel = 0.5–1.0 microns × 90 nm (l, d)
11. Size of hydroxyapatite crystals of dentin = 100 nm × 3 nm (l, d) crystals of dentin = 300 times smaller than of enamel (100 × 3 nm)
12. When 1 mm^2 of dentin is exposed then =30,000 cells are damaged.
13. Specific gravity of enamel = 2.8
14. Rate of enamel formation = 5.0 micron / day.
15. Rate of dentin formation =10–1 5 micron / day.
16. Rate of dentin formation when tooth reaches occlusion = 4 micron/day.
17. Rate of dentin formation during repair =1.0 micron / day.

	Inorganic	Organic + H_2O
Enamel	96%	4%
Dentin	65%	35%
Cementum	45 – 50 %	50 – 55 %
Bone	65%	35%

12

MCQs in Dental Anatomy and Histology

1. Bilateral contraction of the posterior fibers of the temporalis muscles results in which mandibular movement listed below?

A. Retrusion
B. Protrusion
C. Opening
D. Closing

2. How does the distoincisal angle of most anterior teeth compare to the mesioincisal angle?

A. It is straighter
B. It is more rounded
C. There is no difference
D. None of the above

3. All of the following teeth are non-succedaneous, except:

A. The permanent maxillary and mandibular premolars
B. The permanent maxillary and mandibular first molars
C. The permanent maxillary and mandibular second molars
D. The permanent maxillary and mandibular third molars

4. What percentage of dentin is organic?

A. 5-10%
B. 20%

C. 30%
D. 60%

5. **Which primary mandibular tooth listed below does not resemble any other primary or permanent tooth?**
A. Primary mandibular canine
B. Primary mandibular lateral incisor
C. Primary mandibular first molar
D. Primary mandibular second molar

6. **The triangular space between adjacent teeth cervical to the contact area is called as:**
A. Dead space
B. Freeway space
C. Interproximal space
D. Inter-radicular space

7. **The chewing surface of posterior teeth is referred to as the:**
A. Anatomic crown
B. Clinical crown
C. Incisal edge
D. Occlusal surface

8. **Gingival fibers are found within the:**
A. Attached and free gingiva
B. Attached gingiva
C. Free gingiva
D. Mucogingival junction

9. **Which tooth listed below is very often a developmental anomaly with only a slight resemblance to other permanent teeth?**
A. Maxillary first molar
B. Mandibular second molar
C. Maxillary third molar
D. Mandibular first premolar

10. **When viewed from the mesial or distal, mandibular molar crowns appear to be**
A. Tilted buccally
B. Tilted lingually
C. Straight
D. None of the above

11. **During typical empty mouth swallowing, the mandible is braced in which jaw position below to allow for proper stabilization?**
    A. Centric relation (CR)
    B. Intercuspal position (ICP)
    C. Retruded contact position (RCP)
    D. Protruded contact position (PCP)

12. **Which of the following teeth may have a pulp chamber that will be triangular?**
    A. Permanent mandibular second premolars
    B. Permanent maxillary molars
    C. Permanent maxillary lateral incisors
    D. Permanent mandibular canines

13. **In an ideal intercuspal position, the mesiobuccal cusp of the permanent maxillary second molar opposes what?**
    A. The buccal groove of the mandibular second molar
    B. The developmental-groove between the distobuccal and distal cusps of the mandibular first molar
    C. The distobuccal groove of the mandibular first molar
    D. The mesiobuccal groove of the mandibular second molar
    E. The mesiobuccal groove of the mandibular first molar

14. **The lateral pterygoid muscles help perform which two mandibular movements listed below?**
    A. Closing
    B. Opening
    C. Retrusion
    D. Protrusion

15. **The mandible functions as which type of lever?**
    A. Class I
    B. Class II
    C. Class III
    D. Class IV

16. **In the early stage of lateral movement, the condyle appears to rotate with a slight lateral shift in the direction of the movement. This movement is called the Bennett movement and it refers to the:**
    A. Non- working side condyle only

B. Working side condyle only
C. Both the nonworking and working side condyles
D. None of the above

17. Which tooth listed below may have a pulp chamber that is somewhat triangular as opposed to oval
A. Maxillary central incisor
B. Mandibular central incisor
C. Maxillary lateral incisor
D. Mandibular lateral incisor

18. The primary maxillary canine typically erupts around what age?
A. 7 months old
B. 10 month old
C. 18 month old
D. 24 month old

19. The character of occlusal contacts in the unworn dental arch are all of the following except:
A. Point-to-Point
B. Edge-to-edge
C. Edge-to-area
D. Area-to-area

20. The pulp is composed of:
A. Loose connective tissue (collagen and reticulin fibers)
B. Cells (fibroblasts, odontoblasts, histocytes, and lymphocytes)
C. Blood vessels (arteries and veins)
D. Nerves
E. Lymphatic
F. Ground substance
G. All of the above

21. Which of the following is the main function of cementum?
A. Compensation for tooth wear
B. Reparative
C. To attach the principal fibers of the periodontal ligament to the tooth
D. Protection

22. Which primary mandibular molar listed below has a prominent transverse ridge that unites the mesiobuccal and mesiolingual cusps?
   A. Primary mandibular first molar
   B. Primary mandibular second molar
   C. Primary maxillary first molar
   D. Primary maxillary second molar

23. What is the minimum number of lobes from which any tooth may develop?
   A. Two
   B. Three
   C. Four
   D. Five

24. All posterior teeth have how many line angles?
   A. Two
   B. Four
   C. Six
   D. Eight

25. All of the following statements concerning the mandibular lateral incisor are true, except:
   A. The mandibular lateral incisor is a little larger in all dimensions than the mandibular central incisor
   B. The crown of the mandibular lateral incisor is not as bilaterally symmetrical as the mandibular central incisor
   C. The cingulum is directly in the center of the lingual surface
   D. The root is very narrow mesiodistally

26. Oversized anomalies are more common with which tooth listed below?
   A. Maxillary third molar
   B. Mandibular third molar
   C. Mandibular second premolars
   D. Maxillary first molars

27. The excessive formation of cementum around the root of a tooth after it has erupted is known as:
   A. Gomphosis
   B. Ankylosis

C. Hypercementosis
D. Osteodontosis

28. Occlusocervically, the height of the distal marginal ridge of a permanent maxillary first molar is the same height as:
A. The distal marginal ridge of a permanent maxillary second premolar
B. The mesial marginal ridge of a permanent mandibular first molar
C. The mesial marginal ridge of a permanent maxillary second molar
D. The mesial marginal ridge of a permanent maxillary second premolar

29. Drug with teratogenic effects can produce:
A. An abnormal fetus
B. Hyperglycemia
C. Renal toxicity
D. Tumors

30. In an ideal intercuspal position, the facial cusp tips of permanent maxillary premolars oppose what?
A. The facial embrasure between their class counterpart and the tooth mesial to it
B. The facial embrasure between their class counterpart and the tooth distal to it
C. The opposing central fossae
D. The opposing mesial marginal ridge

31. All of the following types of oral mucosa are non-keratinized except:
A. Buccal mucosa
B. Inferior surface of the tongue
C. The soft palate
D. Floor of the mouth
E. Hard palate

32. Of the choices listed below, which one describes the boundaries that define the attached gingiva?
A. From the gingival margin to the interdental groove
B. From the free gingival groove to the gingival margin

C. From the mucogingival junction to the free gingival groove
D. From the epithelial attachment to the cementoenamel junction

33. The mesial and distal aspect (or surfaces) of all anterior teeth have a
A. Trapezoidal outline
B. Triangular outline
C. Square outline
D. Oval shape

34. Which of the following are the three cardinal rules regarding the eruption of teeth
A. Boys before girls
B. Girls before boys
C. Maxillary before mandibular
D. Mandibular before maxillary
E. Slender before stocky
F. Stocky before slender

35. On the lingual surface of all maxillary and mandibular posterior teeth, the height of contour (crest of curvature) is located in the:
A. Occlusal third
B. Middle third
C. Cervical third
D. Gingival third

36. Ordinarily, a 6-year-old child would have what teeth clinically visible in the mouth?
A. All (20) primary teeth and 4 permanent first molars
B. 18 Primary teeth and 2 permanent mandibular central incisors
C. 18 primary teeth, 2 permanent mandibular central incisors and 4 permanent first molars.
D. None of the above

37. Which of the following is the main function of the dental pulp?
A. Nutritive
B. Sensory
C. Protective
D. Formative

38. Which of the following is formed very rapidly in response to irritants?
A. Primary dentin
B. Secondary dentin
C. Reparative dentin
D. Sclerotic dentin

39. Which statement below is *true?*
A. The sum of the mesiodistal widths of the *primary molars* in any one quadrant is equal to the permanent teeth that succeed them *(premolars)*
B. The sum of the mesiodistal widths of the *Primary Molars* in any one quadrant is less than the permanent teeth succeed them *(premolars)*
C. The sum of the mesiodistal widths of the *Primary Molars* in any one quadrant is *greater than* the permanent teeth that succeed them (premolars)
D. None of the above

40. The difference b/w the sum of MD widths of primary c, d, e teeth and that of permanent 3, 4, 5 teeth is known as?
A. Free way space
B. Lee way space of Nance
C. Inter-occlusal distance
D. E – space

41. The distance b/w the occlusal surfaces of upper arch and lower arch at rest position is called as:
A. Free way space
B. Lee way space
C. E – space
D. None of the above

42. A *mesiolingual* developmental groove is a positive ID for which tooth listed below?
A. Maxillary first premolar
B. Mandibular first premolar
C. Maxillary second premolar
D. Mandibular second premolar

43. Which tooth listed below is the *most stable* and self-cleansing?
A. Mandibular central incisor
B. Mandibular first premolar
C. Maxillary canine
D. Maxillary lateral incisor

44. A *small elevation of enamel* found on the crown portion of a tooth would be classified as what?
A. Tubercle
B. Mamelon
C. Ridge
D. Developmental depression

45. The lobes of anterior teeth are always separated by which of the following?
A. Sulci
B. Developmental depressions
C. Inclined planes
D. Developmental artefact

46. Which cusp on permanent maxillary molars generally is the one that gets progressively smaller as you go posterior in the arch?
A. Mesiobuccal
B. Distobuccal
C. Mesiolingual
D. Distolingual

47. The wearing away of tooth structure by mechanical means is known as:
A. Attrition
B. Erosion
C. Abrasion
D. Ablation

48. The mandibular molars have a decided inclination in which direction?
A. Facially
B. Lingually
C. Neither facially or lingually
D. Distally

49. Caries is usually found on all of the following areas, except:
A. Proximal surfaces
B. Pits and grooves
C. Cusp tips
D. Cervical thirds

50. In the intercuspal position, *the distobuccal cusp of a permanent* mandibular first molar occludes where?
A. The interproximal marginal ridge between maxillary second bicuspid and first molar
B. Central fossa of the maxillary first molar
C. Central fossa of the maxillary second molar
D. The interproximal marginal ridge area between maxillary first molar and second molar

51. Which permanent teeth listed below occlude with only one tooth in the opposite jaw assuming that an ideal relation ship exists?
A. Maxillary canines
B. Maxillary central incisors
C. Mandibular central incisors
D. Mandibular third molars

52. Which component of the free gingiva listed below fills the embrasure space between the area of tooth contact?
A. Free gingival groove
B. Gingival sulcus
C. Interdental gingiva
D. Gingival margin

53. Which group of gingival fibers listed below resists rotational forces that are applied to a tooth?
A. Trans-septal fibers
B. Dento-gingival fibers
C. Alveolo-gingival fibers
D. Circumferential fibers
E. Dentoperiosteal fibers

54. Which teeth listed below typically have trifurcations?
A. Mandibular molars
B. Maxillary molars

C. Mandibular premolars
D. Maxillary first premolars

55. On a maxillary molar the largest, longest and strongest of the three roots is the
A. Mesiobuccal
B. Distobuccal
C. Palatal
D. Mesiolingual

56. When a mandibular movement to the left is performed, which condyle moves anteriorly, downward and medially, and also rotates at the same time?
A. Working condyle (left)
B. Nonworking condyle (right)
C. Both of the above
D. Nothing happens

57. When do the deciduous (primary) teeth begin to form in utero?
A. One week
B. Three week
C. Six weeks
D. Ten weeks

58. Which stage in the life cycle of a tooth listed below includes final shaping of the tooth?
A. Initiation (Bud stage)
B. Proliferation (Cap stage)
C. Differentiation (Bell stage)
D. Apposition

59. Which of the following cells form cementum?
A. Ameloblasts
B. Cementoblasts
C. Cementoclasts
D. Odontoblasts

60. Which teeth listed below when viewed from the facial resemble a pentagon (five-sided)?
A. Canines
B. Centrals

C. Laterals
D. Molars

61. Which of the following are primary centers of calcification?
A. Ridges
B. Lobes
C. Grooves
D. Pearls

62. Any linear elevation on the surface of a tooth is called what?
A. An incline
B. A prominence
C. A ridge
D. A tuberosity

63. Which tooth listed below is most often restored, extracted, or replaced
A. Maxillary first molar
B. Mandibular first molar
C. Mandibular first premolar
D. Maxillary first premolar

64. Which maxillary premolar listed below is distinguished by having many accessory grooves on the occlusal surface?
A. First premolar
B. Second premolar
C. Both of the above
D. None of the above

65. As a general rule, root tips tend to curve which way
A. Towards the mesial
B. Towards the distal
C. Towards the mesial on maxillary teeth and toward the distal on mandibular teeth
D. Toward the distal on maxillary teeth and toward the mesial on mandibular teeth

66. The term "homodont" means what?
A. Teeth are continually being replaced
B. Teeth differ from one another
C. Teeth are all alike
D. Long teeth

67. How does mandibular arch generally compare in length with the maxillary arch?

A. It is exactly the same
B. It is slightly longer
C. It is slightly shorter
D. None of the above

68. In the intercuspal position, the mesiolingual cusp of a permanent maxillary second molar occludes where?

A. Central fossa of the mandibular first molar
B. Central fossa of the mandibular second molar
C. The interproximal marginal ridge areas between the mandibular first and second molars
D. The interproximal marginal ridge areas between the mandibular second and third molars

69. All of the following statements concerning supporting cusps are true, except

A. They contact the opposing tooth in the intercuspal position
B. They support the vertical dimension of the face
C. They are nearer the facio-lingual center of the tooth than the non-supporting cusps
D. Their outer incline has a potential for contact
E. They have narrower and sharper cusp ridges than non-supporting cusps

70. In the absence of periodontal disease, the configurations of the crest of the interdental alveolar septa are determined by which of the following?

A. The relative positions of the contact points between teeth
B. The relative positions of the adjacent cementoenamel junctions
C. The relative positions of the heights of contour between adjacent teeth
D. None of the above

71. Which group listed below of the principle fibers of the periodontal ligament runs perpendicular from the alveolar bone to the cementum and resists lateral forces?

A. Alveolar crest

B. Horizontal
C. Oblique
D. Apical

72. The cemento- enamel junction (cervical line) of teeth curves in which two directions?
A. Towards the apex on the facial and lingual surfaces
B. Away from the apex on the facial and lingual surfaces
C. Towards the apex on the mesial and distal surface
D. Away from the apex on the mesial and distal surfaces

73. How many planes of movement can the mandible move in ?
A. One
B. Two
C. Three
D. Four

74. The connective tissue between the cementum of a tooth and the alveolar bone is called the
A. Gingival sulcus
B. Periodontal ligament
C. Periosteum
D. Pulp

75. All of the following are characteristics common to all mandibular anterior teeth, except:
A. Indistinct cingula with smooth lingual anatomy without grooves and pits
B. Incisal edges are lingual to the root axis line
C. The facial surfaces are marked by pronounced labial ridges
D. Continuous convexity inciso-apically on the facial surface

76. A maxillary right canine may be distinguished from a maxillary left canine because
A. The root always curves to the distal in the apical one-third.
B. The distal half of the canine shows more convexity than the mesial half.
C. Labially, the cusp tip is placed distal to a line which bisects the crown and root.
D. Lingually, the cervical line slopes mesially.

77. Of the two mandibular incisors, which has a root that is larger in all dimensions?

A. Mandibular central incisor
B. Mandibular lateral incisor
C. Both have equal roots
D. None of the above

78. Which cusp ridge listed below is longest on the permanent canines?

A. Labial
B. Lingual
C. Mesial
D. Distal

79. Which of the following is the fundamental morphologic unit of enamel?

A. Enamel tuft
B. Enamel spindle
C. Enamel rod
D. Enamel lamellae

80. All of the following statements are true, except:

A. The primary teeth are darker in color than the permanent teeth
B. The pulp cavities are proportionately large in the primary teeth
C. In general, the crowns of primary teeth are more bulbous and constricted than the permanent counterpart
D. The crown surface of all primary teeth are much smoother than the permanent teeth (in other words, there is less evidence of pits and grooves)

81. A sharply defined, shallow, linear depression formed during tooth development which usually separates the primary parts of the crown is called a:

A. Supplemental groove
B. Developmental groove
C. Transverse ridge
D. Triangular ridge

82. Any union of two triangular ridges produces a single ridge, which is called as:

A. A cusp ridge

B. A marginal ridge
C. A transverse ridge
D. A proximal ridge

83. Part of the free gingiva include all of the following except:
A. Gingival margin
B. Free gingival groove
C. Mucogingival junction
D. Gingival sulcus
E. Interdental (interproximal) gingiva

84. Which tooth listed below is the smallest and the narrowest (mesial to distal) of all permanent teeth?
A. Mandibular central incisor
B. Mandibular lateral incisor
C. Maxillary central incisor
D. Maxillary lateral incisor

85. Which ligament below is the only one that gives direct support to the capsule of the TMJ?
A. Sphenomandibular ligament
B. Stylohyoid ligament
C. Stylomandibular ligament
D. Temporomandibular ligament

86. All of the following muscles are involved in elevating the mandible (closing the mouth), except:
A. Masseter muscles
B. Medial pterygoid muscles
C. Lateral pterygoid muscles
D. Temporalis muscles

87. Rotational movements take place in which compartment of the TMJ?
A. Upper (mandibular fossa-disc) compartment
B. Lower (condyle-disc) compartment
C. Both of the above
D. None of the above

88. Cervical line contours are closely related to the attachment of gingival at the neck of the tooth. The greatest contours of

the cervical lines and gingival attachments occur on which of the following surfaces?

A. Distal surfaces of anterior teeth
B. Distal surfaces of posterior teeth
C. Mesial surfaces of anterior teeth
D. Mesial surfaces of posterior teeth

89. The permanent mandibular lateral incisor typically erupts around what age?

A. 5 Years old
B. 7 Years old
C. 10 Years old
D. 12 Years old

90. The distal contact area of a permanent mandibular canine is usually located where?

A. Incisal third
B. Middle third
C. Junction of the incisal and middle third
D. None of the above

91. The tooth germ is composed of all the three structures listed below except?

A. Enamel organ
B. Dental sac
C. Dental papilla
D. Hertwig's epithelial root sheath

92. Which structure listed below is the first formed by the tooth germ and remains in evidence in the formed tooth?

A. Cemento-enamel junction (CEJ)
B. Dentino-enamel junction (DEJ)
C. Cemento-dentinal junction (CDJ)
D. Mucogingival junction (MGJ)

93. For every contact area there are how many embrasures?

A. One
B. Two
C. Three
D. Four

94. "Primate spaces" in the primary dentition are found in which two locations?

A. In the, maxillary arch, the primate space is located between the central incisors and lateral incisors
B. In the maxillary arch, the primate space is located between the lateral incisors and canines
C. In the mandibular arch, the primate space is located between the canines and first molars
D. In the mandibular arch, the primate space is located between the lateral incisors and canines

95. The temporomandibular joint is which type of joint?

A. Hinge joint
B. Gliding (sliding) joint
C. Combined hinge and gliding (sliding) joint
D. None of the above

96. Which of the following molars is the most symmetrical?

A. Maxillary second molar
B. Maxillary first molar
C. Mandibular first molar
D. Mandibular second molar

97. Which anterior tooth listed below is most likely to have a bifurcated root?

A. Maxillary central incisor
B. Mandibular canine
C. Mandibular incisor
D. Maxillary canine

98. How many root are visible from the buccal aspect of a maxillary first molar?

A. One roots
B. Two roots
C. Three roots
D. Four

99. A child with an anterior open bite of the moderate severity should be presumed to have what habit until proven otherwise?

A. Mouth breathing

B. Thumb sucking
C. Pencil biting
D. Night time milk drinking

100. Which tooth listed below has a mesial marginal ridge that is distinctly shorter in length and less prominent in height than the distal marginal ridge?
A. Maxillary first molar
B. Mandibular first premolar
C. Mandibular second premolar
D. Maxillary canine

101. Which premolar listed below is the only one that has a mesial buccal cusp ridge that is longer than its distal buccal cusp ridge?
A. Maxillary first premolar
B. Maxillary second premolar
C. Mandibular first premolar
D. Mandibular second premolar

102. All of the muscles are considered to be extrinsic muscles of the tongue except:
A. Genioglossus muscle
B. Longitudinal muscle
C. Hyoglossus muscle
D. Palatoglossus muscle

103. The surfaces of which teeth listed below have a trapezoid outline?
A. Lingual and labial of posterior teeth
B. Lingual and facial of all teeth
C. Proximal surfaces of anterior teeth
D. Proximal surfaces of all posterior teeth

104. All of the following are the theoretical determinants needed for restoring a complete and functional occlusal surface of a tooth except:
A. The amount of vertical overlap of the anterior teeth
B. The contour of the articular eminence
C. The amount and direction of lateral shift in the working side condyle

D. The position of the tooth in the arch
E. The height of the pulp horn of that particular tooth.

105. When posterior teeth are in a normal ideal relationship, which of the following cusps are considered to be supporting cusps?
A. Maxillary lingual cusps
B. Maxillary buccal cusps
C. Mandibular lingual cusps
D. Mandibular buccal cusps
E. All of the above

106. Which succedaneous teeth are usually the last to erupt?
A. Maxillary canines
B. Mandibular canines
C. Mandibular second premolars
D. None of the above

107. When the mandible is in its physiologic rest or postural position, contact of teeth is :
A. Maximum
B. Not present
C. Premature
D. Slight

108. Which of the following decreases with age in the dental pulp?
A. Number of collagen fibers
B. Number of reticulin fibers
C. The size of the pulp
D. Calcifications within the pulp

109. The permanent mandibular first molar has a morphology closely resembles which primary tooth listed below?
A. Primary mandibular first molar
B. Primary mandibular second molar
C. Primary maxillary first molar
D. None of the above

110. Which of the following encloses the TMJ like a tube?
A. Bowman's capsule
B. Crosby capsule

C. Fibrous capsule
D. Glisson's capsule

111. A diarthrodial joint is:
A. A joint that permits no movement at all
B. A joint that permits relatively free movement
C. Joint that permits slight movement
D. None of the above

112. Which permanent tooth listed below (other than the third molars) varies in form more than any other tooth?
A. Maxillary centrals
B. Mandibular centrals
C. Maxillary laterals
D. Mandibular lateral

113. Which tooth below may show three types of occlusal surfaces?
A. Maxillary first premolar
B. Mandibular second premolar
C. Mandibular first premolar
D. Maxillary second premolar

114. Which premolar listed below is usually the largest?
A. Maxillary first
B. Maxillary second
C. Mandibular first
D. Mandibular second

115. All of the following muscles are infrahyoid muscles, except the:
A. Thyrohyoid muscle
B. Sternohyoid muscle
C. Omohyoid muscle
D. Mylohyoid muscle
E. Sternothyroid muscle

116. Which of the following is a hereditary dental defect in which the enamel of the teeth is soft and undercalcified in context, yet of normal quantity?
A. Enamel hypoplasia

B. Enamel hypocalcification
C. Fluorosis
D. Enamel hypomaturation

117. Which muscle listed below plays a subsidiary role in mastication?
A. Masseter
B. Lateral pterygoid
C. Buccinator
D. Medial pterygoid
E. Temporalis

118. If a maxillary first molar has a fourth canal, it will be located where?
A. In the palatal root
B. In the distobuccal root
C. In the mesiobuccal root
D. In the distal furcation

119. The determinants of occlusion include
A. The right temporomandibular joint and its suspensory ligaments
B. The left temporomandibular joint and its suspensory ligaments
C. The occlusal surfaces of the teeth
D. The neuromuscular system
E. All of the above

120. In an ideal intercuspal position, the mesiolingual cusps of permanent mandibular molars oppose what?
A. The opposing central fossae
B. The lingual embrasure between their class counterpart and the tooth distal to it
C. The opposing distal marginal ridge
D. The lingual embrasure between their class counterpart and the tooth mesial to it

121. The periodontium includes
A. The gingiva
B. The periodontal ligament
C. The cementum

D. The alveolar and supporting bone
E. All of the above

122. All of the following anterior teeth have a cingulum which is located in the center of the lingual surface, except:
A. Maxillary lateral incisor
B. Mandibular canine
C. Maxillary canine
D. Mandibular central incisor

123. The permanent maxillary canine is most likely to occlude with which of the following mandibular teeth?
A. Lateral incisor and canine
B. Canine only
C. Canine and first premolar
D. First premolar only

124. When viewed from a buccal or lingual aspect the crowns of all mandibular and maxillary incisors appear to have a :
A. Triangular outline
B. Trapezoidal outline
C. Rhomboidal outline
D. Rectangular outline

125. Which of the following is the first deciduous (primary) tooth to erupt?
A. Mandibular central incisor
B. Mandibular first molar
C. Maxillary central incisor
D. Maxillary first molar

126. Which of the following is the hardest substance in the body?
A. Enamel
B. Dentin
C. Cementum
D. Bone

127. All of the following are the four distinct layers of the enamel organ except?
A. Outer enamel epithelium
B. Inner enamel epithelium

C. Stratum granulosum
D. Stratum intermedium
E. Stellate reticulum

128. Mamelons are found on newly erupting
A. Molars
B. Canines
C. Premolars
D. Incisors

129. Which ridge listed below is found only on maxillary molars?
A. Labial ridge
B. Marginal ridge
C. Oblique ridge
D. Transverse ridge

130. The periodontal ligament is made up of all of the following except:
A. Collagenous fibers
B. Nerves
C. Lymphatics
D. Blood vessels
E. Cartilages

131. The roots of all but one anterior are likely to have longitudinal grooves on the mesial and distal surfaces. Which tooth listed below doesn't have these grooves?
A. Maxillary canine
B. Maxillary lateral incisor
C. Maxillary central incisor
D. Mandibular lateral incisor

132. Which tooth listed below has a small DL cusp that can be absent, creating a three-cups tooth?
A. Mandibular second molar
B. Maxillary first molar
C. Mandibular first premolar
D. Maxillary second molar

133. A fissured groove is most frequently found on which surface listed below
A. Facial of maxillary molars

B. Lingual of maxillary molars
C. Facial of mandibular molars
D. Lingual of mandibular molars

134. During working side movement of the mandible, the oblique ridge of a maxillary first molar passes through which sulcus listed below of a permanent mandibular first molar?
A. Mesiobuccal sulcus
B. Distobuccal sulcus
C. Mesiolingual sulcus
D. Distolingual sulcus

135. The prime mover in effecting a left working-side movements is :
A. The right medial pterygoid muscle
B. The left medial pterygoid muscle
C. The right lateral pterygoid muscle
D. The left lateral pterygoid muscle

136. A patient with a paralyzed right lateral pterygoid muscle is instructed to open his mouth wide. Which direction will the mandible deviates to upon opening?
A. To the right
B. To the left
C. It will not deviate to right or left
D. None of the above

137. Which of the following terms refers to tooth contacts while the mandibular is in action, such as during mastication and swallowing?
A. Centric relation
B. Centric occlusion
C. Functional occlusion
D. Malocclusion

138. Which three mandibular teeth listed below are so aligned that when viewed from the occlusal, a straight line may be drawn that will bisect all contact areas?
A. Central incisor, lateral incisor and canine
B. Canine, first premolar and second premolar
C. Second premolar, first molar, and second molar
D. None of the above

139. A child 19 months old will have how many teeth?

A. Four

B. Eight

C. Twelve

D. Sixteen

E. Twenty

140. When viewed from the facial, all premolars have their contacts where?

A. Middle third

B. Junction of the occlusal and middle third

C. Occlusal third

D. Cervical third

141. Morphologically, the primary maxillary second molar strikingly resembles which permanent tooth listed below?

A. Permanent maxillary third molar

B. Permanent maxillary second molar

C. Permanent maxillary first molar

D. Permanent mandibular second molar

142. Which of the following is the first layer of dentin formed?

A. Mantle dentin

B. Peritubular dentin

C. Intertubular dentin

D. Interglobular dentin

143. A long depression or a V-shaped valley on the occlusal surface of a posterior tooth located between ridge and cusps is called a:

A. Pit

B. Sulcus

C. Fossa

D. Fissure

144. Which primary molar listed below is the most atypical of all the molars, primary and permanent and appears to be intermediate in form and development between a premolar and molar?

A. Primary mandibular first molar

B. Primary maxillary first molar

C. Primary mandibular second molar
D. Primary maxillary second molar

145. What is the term used to describe the triangularly shaped spaces located between the proximal surfaces of adjacent teeth?
A. A contact area
B. An occlusal curvature
C. A gingival space
D. An embrasure

146. The articular disc (meniscus) is a fibrous saddle-shaped structure that separates:
A. The condyle and the sphenoid bone
B. The condyle and the ethmoid bone
C. The condyle and the temporal bone
D. The condyle and the occipital bone

147. The cusp of Carabelli is often on which permanent tooth listed below?
A. Maxillary second molar
B. Maxillary first molar
C. Mandibular first molar
D. Mandibular second molar

148. Which tooth listed below has a mesial development depression?
A. Mandibular first premolar
B. Maxillary second premolar
C. Maxillary first premolar
D. Mandibular second premolar

149. The mental foramen is located most closely to the apex of which tooth listed below?
A. Mandibular canine
B. Mandibular second premolar
C. Mandibular first molar
D. Maxillary first premolar

150. The parotid duct opens on the oral surface of the cheek through a small opening opposite which tooth listed below?
A. Maxillary first premolar

B. Maxillary second molar
C. Mandibular first molar
D. Mandibular second molar

151. Which of the following is a developmental abnormality characterized by the total absence of teeth?
A. Hypodontia
B. Anodontia
C. Diphyodontia
D. Hypsodontia

152. All of the following are suprahyoid muscle, except the :
A. Geniohyoid muscle
B. Mylohyoid muscle
C. Stylohyoid muscle
D. Digastric muscle
E. Omohyoid muscle

153. Which of the following is a hereditary dental defect in which the enamel of the teeth is soft and undercalcified in context yet normal in quantity?
A. Enamel hypoplasia
B. Enamel hypocalcification
C. Fluorosis
D. None of the above

154. Which cusp listed below of the permanent maxillary first molar serves as a reference point in identifying Angle's Class I, II, and III occlusion?
A. Distobuccal
B. Distolingual
C. Mesiobuccal
D. Mesiolingual

155. The periodontal ligament fibers are anchored into cementum and bone by :
A. Gray fibers
B. Purkinje's fibers
C. Sharpey's fibers
D. Spindle fibers

156. Which structure listed below is the inner layer of cells of the junctional epithelium and attaches the gingiva to the tooth?

A. Mucogingival junction
B. Free gingival groove
C. Epithelial attachment
D. Gingival pocket

157. Which of the following provides the most common criterion for differentiating permanent mandibular central incisors from permanent mandibular lateral incisors?

A. Difference in root length
B. Difference in ratio of crown length to root length
C. Degree of slope of the incisal edge when viewed facially
D. Difference in rotation of the crown on the root

158. Which teeth listed below are the only ones have labial ridges?

A. Centrals
B. Laterals
C. Canines
D. Molars

159. The RCP is what type of the position?

A. Tooth guided
B. Ligament guided
C. Muscle guided
D. None of the above

160. The character of occlusal contacts in the unworn dental arch are all of the following except

A. Point-to –Point
B. Point-to-Area
C. Edge-to-edge
D. Edge-to-area
E. Area-to-area

161. A small elevation resulting from overproduction of enamel (enamel pearls) would be classified as what?

A. Cusp
B. Tubercle

C. Mamelon
D. Ridge

162. A pinpoint depression at the junction or terminus of grooves is called what?
A. Fossae
B. Fissure
C. Pit
D. Sulcus

163. In the intercuspal position, the distobuccal cusp of a permanent mandibular first molar occludes where?
A. The interproximal marginal ridge area between maxillary second bicusid and first molar
B. Central fossa of the maxillary first molar
C. Central fossa of the maxillary second molar
D. The interproximal marginal ridge area between maxillary first molar and second molar

164. In the intercuspal position, the mesiolingual cusp of permanent maxillary second molar occludes where?
A. Central fossa of the mandibular first molar
B. Central fossa of the mandibular second molar
C. The interproximal marginal ridge areas between mandibular second and third molars
D. The distal fossa of first molar

165. The axial surfaces of which teeth listed below have a rhomboid outline?
A. Buccal of mandibular posterior teeth
B. Buccal of maxillary posterior teeth
C. Lingual of maxillary posterior teeth
D. Mesial and distal of mandibular posterior teeth
E. Mesial and distal of maxillary posterior teeth

166. All teeth have how many line angles?
A. Two
B. Four
C. Six
D. Eight

167. The divergence of two proximal surfaces from the area of contact, facially, lingually, occlusally, and gingivally, creates a space, which is called as?

A. A contact area
B. A gingival space
C. An embrasure
D. An occlusal curvature

168. The primary first molar is usually exfoliated between what ages?

A. 6-8 years
B. 7-9 years
C. 10-12 years
D. 12-14 years

169. A primary centre of growth or calcification on a tooth is called what?

A. Lobe
B. Ridge
C. Cingulum
D. Groove

170. The interproximal space is a triangular area. The base and the sides of this triangle are represented by which of the following?

A. Buccal embrasure
B. Lingual
C. Alveolar bone
D. Proximal surfaces of the teeth
E. Occlusal embrasure

171. The height of contour are located where on the lingual surface of all maxillary molars?

A. Occlusal third
B. Middle third
C. Cervical third
D. None of the above

172. When viewed from the facial, all molars have their contacts where?

A. Middle third

B. Junction of the occlusal and middle third
C. Occlusal third
D. All of the above

173. Which of the following cusps are referred to as "stamp cusps"?
A. Maxillary lingual cusps
B. Maxillary buccal cusps
C. Mandibular lingual cusps
D. Mandibular buccal cusps

174. When posterior teeth are in normal ideal relationship, which of the following cusps are considered supporting cusps?
A. Maxillary lingual
B. Maxillary facial
C. Mandibular lingual
D. Mandibular facial

175. Which mandibular deciduous tooth does not resemble any permanent tooth?
A. Deciduous canine
B. Deciduous lateral
C. Deciduous first molar
D. Deciduous second molar

176. Which primary molar listed below is the most atypical of all the molars, primary and permanent, and appears to be intermediate in form and development between a premolar and a molar
A. Mandibular first primary molar
B. Maxillary first primary molar
C. Mandibular second primary molar
D. Maxillary second primary molar

177. Name two ridges which are present on all teeth.
A. Triangular ridges
B. Mesial and distal cusp ridges
C. Oblique ridge
D. Mesial and distal marginal ridges
E. Buccal ridge

178. The surfaces of which teeth listed below have a triangular outline?

A. Mesial and distal of anterior teeth
B. Mesial and distal of posterior maxillary teeth
C. Mesial and distal of posterior mandibular teeth
D. Labial of anterior teeth
E. Lingual of anterior teeth

179. Which of the following provides the most reliable criterion for differentiating permanent mandibular central incisors from permanent mandibular lateral incisors?

A. Difference in root length
B. Difference in ratio of crown length to root length
C. Degree of slope of the incisal edge when viewed facially
D. Difference in rotation of the crown on the root

180. The cingulum of most anterior teeth is located where?

A. In the centre of the lingual surface.
B. In the mesial portion of the lingual surface.
C. In the distal portion of the lingual surface.
D. Near the incisal edges of the teeth

181. Oversized anomalies are more common with which tooth listed below?

A. Maxillary third molar
B. Mandibular third molar
C. Maxillary premolars
D. Mandibular lateral incisors

182. The only anterior tooth which occasionally shows three developmental depressions on its labial surface is which of the following?

A. Maxillary central
B. Maxillary lateral
C. Maxillary cuspid
D. Mandibular cuspid
E. Mandibular lateral

183. Which of the premolars is usually the largest?

A. Maxillary first
B. Maxillary second

C. Mesial surface of anterior teeth
D. Mandibular second

184. A mesiolingual developmental groove is a positive ID for what tooth?
A. Maxillary first premolar
B. Mandibular first premolar
C. Maxillary second premolar
D. Mandibular second premolar

185. The region of the pulp that is relatively cell poor is called what?
A. Coronal pulp
B. Zone of Weil
C. Radicular pulp
D. Central zone

186. Lobes of teeth are usually separated by which of the following?
A. Depressions
B. Developmental grooves
C. Sulci
D. Depressions or developmental groove
E. Developmental groove or sulci

187. A linear elevation on the surface of a tooth is called what?
A. Incline
B. Prominence
C. Ridge
D. Tuberosity

188. The wearing away of the incisal or occlusal surfaces is referred to as?
A. Erosion
B. Attrition
C. Abrasion
D. Ablation

189. The largest embrasure associated with the adjacent teeth in contact is which of the following?
A. Occlusal

B. Labial
C. Lingual
D. Buccal

190. What is the minimum number of lobes from which any tooth may develop?
A. Two
B. Three
C. Four
D. Five

191. What is the percentages of dentin that is inorganic?
A. 2-5%
B. 10-15%
C. 20-30%
D. 50-60%
E. 70-80%

192. Give the name for the curve, which runs in a mesial-distal direction along the cusps of lower teeth?
A. Curve of Wilson
B. Curve of Spee
C. Curve of Monson
D. None of the above

193. The gingiva is normally attached to the tooth by what structure?
A. Frenum
B. Epithelial attachment
C. Free gingiva
D. Attached gingiva

194. Which of the following listed below gives rise to the cementum and the periodontal ligament?
A. Dental sac
B. Enamel reticulum
C. Dental papilla
D. Enamel organ

195. Which of these terms describes the tissue formed in response to irritational stimuli produced by carious or mechanical penetration of a tooth?
A. Primary dentin
B. Secondary dentin
C. Dead tracts
D. Sclerotic dentin

196. The primary function of the dental pulp is to:
A. Respond to irritation by its inflammatory reaction
B. Furnish nutrition to the tooth
C. Form dentin
D. Provide sensation

197. What is the fundamental morphological unit of enamel?
A. Enamel prism
B. Enamel tufts
C. Enamel spindles
D. Enamel lamellae

198. What is the percentage of water in fully development enamel?
A. 4%
B. 10%
C. 50%
D. 70%

199. A freely movable joint in which contiguous bony surfaces are covered by articular cartilage and connected by ligaments lined with synovial membrane is referred to as what type joint?
A. Amphi-arthroidal
B. Synarthroidal
C. Diarthroidal
D. None of the above

200. Of the choices listed below, one describes the boundaries that define the attached gingiva?
A. Form the gingival crest to the interdental groove
B. From the free gingival groove to the gingival crest
C. From the mucogingival junction to the free gingival groove

D. From the epithelial attachment to the cementoenamel junction

201. Which tooth listed below has a mesial development depression?

A. Mandibular first premolar
B. Maxillary second premolar
C. Maxillary first premolar
D. Mandibular second premolar

202. When a mandibular movement to the left is performed, which condyle moves anteriorly, downward and medially, and also rotates at the same time?

A. Working condyle (left)
B. Nonworking condyle (right)
C. Both the condyles
D. No movement at all as said above

203. A patient with a paralyzed left genioglossus muscle is instructed to bring his tongue out. Which direction will be tongue take on opening?

A. To the right
B. To the left
C. Straight
D. Downwards

204. Constriction of the posterior fibers of the temporalis muscle results in what mandibular movement?

A. Retrusion
B. Protrusion
C. Opening with translation
D. Closing

205. The combined pull of the two lateral pterygoid muscles along with the anterior bellies of the two digastric and other suprahyoid muscles will result in what mandibular movement?

A. Protrusion
B. Retrusion
C. Closing
D. Opening

206. When the mandible is in its physiologic rest or postural position, contact of teeth is:

A. Maximum
B. Not present
C. Premature
D. Slight

207. Which of the following will have a pulp chamber that will be triangular?

A. Permanent mandibular second premolar
B. Permanent mandibular molars
C. Permanent maxillary molars
D. Permanent maxillary lateral incisors

208. Occlusocervically, the height of the distal marginal ridge of a permanent maxillary first molar is at the same height as which of the following listed below?

A. Mesial marginal ridge of a maxillary second premolar
B. Mesial marginal ridge of a mandibular first molar
C. Mesial marginal ridge of a maxillary second molar
D. Distal marginal ridge of a maxillary second premolar

209. The permanent maxillary canine is most likely to occlude with which of the following mandibular teeth?

A. Lateral incisor and canine
B. Canine only
C. Canine and first premolar
D. First premolar and second premolar.

210. Which of the following muscles is the prime mover in effecting a right working movement?

A. Right lateral pterygoid
B. Right medial pterygoid
C. Left lateral pterygoid
D. Left medial pterygoid

211. Which position listed is one in which there is a relative muscular equilibrium?

A. Retruded contact position
B. Postural position

C. Protruded contact position
D. Intercuspal position

212. Which tooth below may show three types of occlusal surfaces?
A. Maxillary first premolar
B. Mandibular second premolar
C. Mandibular first premolar
D. Maxillary second premolar

213. Which of the following teeth has a mesial marginal ridge that is distinctly shorter in length and less prominent in height than the distal marginal ridge?
A. Maxillary first molar
B. Mandibular first premolar
C. Mandibular first molar
D. Maxillary first premolar

214. The smallest permanent tooth and the narrowest mesial to distal width, is which tooth?
A. Mandibular central incisor
B. Mandibular lateral incisor
C. Maxillary lateral incisor
D. Mandibular canine

215. The roots of all but one anterior tooth are likely to have longitudinal grooves on the mesial and distal surfaces, which tooth doesn't have these grooves?
A. Maxillary canine
B. Maxillary lateral incisor
C. Maxillary central incisor
D. Mandibular lateral incisor

216. A maxillary right canine may be distinguished from a maxillary left canine because:
A. The root always curves to the distal in the apical one-third
B. The distal half of the canine shows more convexity than the mesial half
C. Labially, the cusp tip is placed distal to a line which bisects the crown and root.
D. Lingually, the cervical line slopes mesially.

217. Pits in the occlusal surfaces of molars and premolars are at the junction of which of the following?

A. Marginal ridges and inclined planes
B. Inclined planes and cusp tips
C. Developmental grooves
D. Facial and mesial surfaces

218. The surface of a premolar or molar located within the marginal ridges which contact the corresponding surfaces of antagonists during closure of the posterior teeth is called what?

A. Occlusal table
B. Clinical crown
C. Occlusal surface
D. Height of contour

219. Which primary molar has a prominent transverse ridge that unites the mesiofacial and mesiolingual cusps?

A. First primary mandibular molar
B. Second primary mandibular molar
C. First primary maxillary molar
D. Second primary maxillary molar

220. Which teeth listed below should ideally provide the predominant guidance through the full range of movement in lateral mandibular excursions?

A. Premolars
B. First molars
C. Incisors
D. Canines

QUESTIONS FOR BRAIN DIET AND SELF ANSWERING

1. Listed below are the usual events in the histogenesis of a tooth. Place them in their correct sequence (from what happens first to what happens last).

A. Deposition of the first layer of dentin
B. Differentiation of odontoblasts
C. Deposition of the first layer of enamel
D. Elongation of the inner enamel epithelial cells

2. **The axial surfaces of which teeth listed below have a rhomboid outline?**
   A. Mesial and distal of maxillary posterior teeth
   B. Mesial and distal of mandibular posterior teeth
   C. Lingual of maxillary posterior teeth
   D. Buccal of maxillary posterior teeth
   E. Buccal of mandibular posterior teeth

3. **During typical empty mouth swallowing, the mandible is braced in what position to allow for proper stabilization?**
4. **What is the Bennett movement?**
5. **The vertical overlap of the maxillary incisors to the mandibular incisors is called what?**
6. **What is anterior guidance?**
7. **List four theoretical determinants needed for restoring a complete and functional occlusal surface of a tooth.**
8. **List the four features of the human dentition, which directly affect the health of the periodontal ligament and its hard tissue anchorage in term of resisting occlusal force?**
9. **Which are the basic principles for occlusal adjustment?**
10. **How does the maxillary alveolar bone differs from the mandibular bone?**

Answer Key to MCQs in Dental Anatomy and Histology

1	A	2	B	3	A	4	B
5	C	6	C	7	D	8	C
9	C	10	B	11	B	12	B
13	A	14	B, D	15	C	16	B
17	A	18	C	19	D	20	G
21	C	22	A	23	C	24	D
25	C	26	B	27	C	28	C
29	A	30	B	31	E	32	C
33	B	34	B, D, E	35	B	36	A
37	D	38	C	39	C	40	B
41	A	42	B	43	C	44	A
45	B	46	D	47	C	48	B
49	C	50	B	51	C	52	C
53	D	54	B	55	C	56	B
57	C	58	C	59	B	60	A
61	B	62	C	63	B	64	B
65	B	66	C	67	C	68	B
69	E	70	B	71	B	72	A
73	C	74	B	75	C	76	B
77	B	78	D	79	C	80	A
81	B	82	C	83	C	84	A
85	D	86	C	87	B	88	C
89	B	90	C	91	D	92	B
93	D	94	C	95	C	96	D
97	B	98	C	99	B	100	B
101	A	102	B	103	B	104	E
105	A, D	106	A	107	B	108	B, C
109	B	110	C	111	B	112	C
113	B	114	A	115	D	116	B
117	C	118	C	119	E	120	D
121	E	122	B	123	C	124	B
125	A	126	A	127	C	128	D
129	C	130	E	131	C	132	D
133	B	134	B	135	C	136	A
137	C	138	C	139	D	140	B
141	C	142	A	143	B	144	B

145	D	146	C	147	B	148	C
149	B	150	B	151	B	152	E
153	B	154	C	155	C	156	C
157	D	158	C	159	B	160	E
161	B	162	C	163	B	164	B
165	D	166	D	167	C	168	C
169	A	170	C	171	B	172	A
173	A, D	174	A	175	C	176	B
177	D	178	A	179	D	180	C
181	B	182	C	183	B	184	B
185	B	186	D	187	C	188	B
189	A	190	C	191	E	192	B
193	B	194	A	195	B	196	C
197	A	198	A	199	C	200	C
201	C	202	B	203	B	204	A
205	D	206	B	207	C	208	C
209	C	210	C	211	B	212	B
213	B	214	A	215	C	216	B
217	C	218	C	219	A	220	D

ADDITIONAL MCQs

Section 1

1. On a maxillary first premolar, longitudinal developmental grooves would probably be noted on which of the following root surfaces?

1. Lingual
2. Mesial
3. Facial
4. Palatal

2. A single tooth which is in premature contact when occluding is probably in:

1. Torsoversion
2. Infraversion
3. Linguoversion
4. Supraversion

3. Which occlusal factor is determined during guiding the mandible into centric relation?

1. Canine rise
2. Degree of overbite
3. Centric prematurity
4. Working interference
5. Balancing interference

4. To determine occlusal harmony of the dentition, which of the following tooth relationships should be evaluated?

A. Overlap
B. Interarch
C. Intra-arch
D. Cusp-to-fossa

1. (a), (b) and (c)
2. (b), (c) and (d)
3. (a), (c) and (d)
4. (a), (c) and (d)
5. All of the above

5. The normal relation of the permanent maxillary first molar to the mandibular arch is established in centric occlusion, when the:

1. Maxillary first molar occludes with mandibular second premolar and first molar.
2. Distal surface of the maxillary first molar is in the same plane as the distal surface of the mandibular first molar.
3. Distofacial cusp of the maxillary first molar falls in the same plane as the distal surface of the mandibular first molar.
4. Mesiolingual cusp of the maxillary first molar falls in the central fossa of the mandibular first molar.

6. Parafunctional occlusal habits cause which of the following?

A. Wear facets
B. Uneven wear patterns
C. Mobile teeth
D. Gingivitis
E. Periodontal pockets

1. (a), (b) and (c)
2. (a), (b) and (e)
3. (b), (c) and (d)
4. (b), (c) and (e)
5. (c), (d) and (e)
6. (d) and (e) only
7. All of the above

7. Dental fluorosis has which of the following characteristics?

1. Dark brown staining
2. White opaque areas of enamel
3. Pitting of the enamel surface
4. All of the above

8. What are the functions of the dental papillae and the dental pulp?

A. Dentin formation
B. Influencing ameloblastic activity
C. Providing nerve and blood supply in teeth
D. Cementum formation

1. (a), (b) and (c)
2. (a), (b) and (d)

3. (a), (c) and (d)
4. (b), (c) and (d)
5. All of the above

9. Proper techniques for electric pulp testing (EPT) includes placing the electrode on:

A. Sound tooth structure
B. Teeth with full castings
C. Teeth that have been dried
D. The occlusal third of crowns

1. (a) and (b)
2. (a) and (c)
3. (a) and (d)
4. (b) and (c)
5. (b) and (d)
6. (c) and (d)

10. Which of the following causes lead to exposure of dentin?

A. Erosion
B. Root planning
C. Dental caries
D. Tooth brush abrasion

1. (a) and (b)
2. (a) and (c)
3. (a) and (d)
4. (b) and (c)
5. (b) and (d)
6. (c) and (d)
7. All of the above

11. What are the hard, smooth, spherical structures attached to root surfaces of permanent molars near their cervical lines:

1. Denticles
2. Cementicles
3. Enamel pearls
4. Bony exostoses
5. Retained primary root fragments

12. Root planing is cumbersome in which of the following areas?

1. Trifurcations of maxillary first molars

2. Mesial surfaces of maxillary premolars
3. Distal surfaces of mandibular third molars
4. Proximal surfaces of mandibular anterior teeth

13. Thickest layer of cementum is found in which of the following parts of a root?
1. Exposed root surface
2. Apical third of the root
3. Middle third of the root
4. Coronal third of the root
5. None of the above

14. Which of the following characterize the roots of a mandibular first molar?
A. The roots curve toward the mesial
B. The distal root is wider faciolingually
C. The root surfaces have longitudinal grooves
D. The distal root is shorter and straighter than the mesial root

15. At cementoenamel junction (CEJ), calculus is difficult to discriminate because
1. Pockets are usually deep at the CEJ
2. Broad contacts at the CEJ prevent access
3. Calculus is granular at the CEJ
4. Root surfaces are convex at the CEJ
5. Anatomic characteristics of the CEJ vary

16. At what age, the bottom of the gingival sulcus in a healthy mouth is found to be positioned apical to the CEJ?
1. Prenatally
2. At 10-20 years of age
3. At 40-60 years of age
4. Just after a permanent tooth has erupted
5. Before the roots of primary teeth are resorbed

Section 2

1. What is the normal pattern for eruption of primary teeth?
1. Maxillary central incisors erupt before mandibular central incisors
2. Maxillary canines erupt before maxillary lateral incisors

3. Maxillary first molars erupt before maxillary canines
4. Mandibular canines erupt before mandibular first molars
5. Mandibular second molars erupt before mandibular first molars

2. Due to parents' lack of knowledge of eruption patterns and of differences between permanent and primary teeth, which of the following might result?

1. A 5-year-old child with no primate spaces
2. A 6-year-old child with rampant caries
3. A 9-year-old child with missing permanent first molars
4. A 11-year-old with crowding of mandibular incisors
5. A 11.6 -year-old with unerupted permanent second molars

3. Why are the facial surfaces of maxillary molars are considered food-retentive?

1. These areas are less self-cleaning
2. Stensen's duct opens just opposite the molars
3. Erupted third molars tighten contact areas
4. At rest, the lips force saliva against the molars
5. The tongue pushes food against the molars during mastication

4. Which of the following premolars present the greatest difficulty in endodontic therapy?

1. Maxillary first
2. Maxillary second
3. Mandibular first
4. Mandibular second

5. Which of the following factors affect shape and size of pulp canals?

A. Age
B. Trauma
C. Attrition
D. Function

1. (a) and (b)
2. (a) and (c)
3. (a) and (d)
4. (b) and (d)
5. All of the above

Section 3

1. Root sensitivity is overcome or reduced when there is formation of:
   1. Cementum
   2. Fluorosis
   3. Cemental tubules
   4. Reparative dentin
   5. A deepened sulcus

2. Why is there hypersensitivity in the cervical area of a tooth often occurs when gingival recession takes place?
   1. Exposed cementum, like exposed bone, is highly sensitive
   2. Dentinal sclerosis due to increased activity of odontoblasts
   3. Dentinal tubules are not adequately protected
   4. Dentinal tubules beneath the area of cementum exposure are increased in number

3. Pits in the occlusal surfaces of buccal teeth are generally found at the junctions:
   1. Marginal ridges and inclined planes
   2. Inclined planes and cusp tips
   3. Facial and mesial surfaces
   4. Developmental grooves

Section 4

1. Which of the following premolars is generally having two separate roots?
   1. Maxillary first
   2. Maxillary second
   3. Mandibular first
   4. Mandibular second

2. What is the defense mechanism in the dentin against invasion of the tubules by bacteria?
   1. Sclerosis of the tubules
   2. Swelling of the tubular walls
   3. Demineralisation of the tubules
   4. Proliferation of the odontoblasts

3. Which of the following teeth most frequently have dens in dente?
1. Maxillary central incisor
2. Maxillary lateral incisor
3. Maxillary third molar
4. Mandibular second premolar
5. Mandibular third molar

4. Transmission of the sensation of contact when teeth are occluding is by which of the following tissues?
1. Dental pulp
2. Periosteum
3. Alveolar bone
4. Attached gingiva
5. Periodontal ligament

5. Excessive heat to a tooth results in pain because:
1. All stimuli to the pulp result in a pain sensation
2. Excessive stimulation of a heat receptor always results in pain
3. Heat receptors in the pulp have a low threshold to pain
4. Blood vessels of the pulp expand and cause strangulation of the tissue

6. Difference between the primary molars and permanent molars is that in the primary molars,
1. Less bulbous crowns
2. More pits and fissures
3. Greater divergence of roots
4. None of the above

7. Calculus at the cementoenamel junction is difficult to discriminate because:
1. Calculus is granular
2. Root surfaces are convex
3. Pockets are usually deep
4. Broad contacts prevent access
5. Anatomic characteristics vary
6. Both (1) and (5) above
7. Both (2) and (4) above

8. Heavy keratinization and absence of taste buds are the features of which type of papillae found on tongue surface?
1. Foliate
2. Filiform
3. Fungiform
4. Circumvallate

9. Which part of the periodontium is least affected by traumatic occlusal forces?
1. Cementum
2. Gingival attachment
3. Apical area of the periodontal ligament
4. Oblique fibers of the periodontal ligament

10. All of the following are found in the case of occlusal trauma except:
1. Loss of alveolar bone
2. Increase in tooth mobility
3. Formation of periodontal pockets
4. Increase in width of the periodontal ligament space

Section 5

1. When a hypertonic sucrose solution is applied to a tooth, the mechanism of pain production that occurs, is most probably related to:
1. Dehydration of dental matrix protein
2. Coagulation of dentinal matrix protein
3. Movement of water out of dentinal tubules
4. Piezoelectric effects on hydroxyapatite crystals

2. Which type of papillae is found in maximum numbers on the human tongue?
1. Foliate
2. Filiform
3. Fungiform
4. Circumvallate

3. Thickest layer of cementum is present on which part of the tooth root?
1. Exposed root surface

2. Apical third of the root
3. Middle third of the root
4. Coronal third of the root
5. None of the above

4. Of the following, the root depression that often can be instrumented from the lingual aspect only is on the mesial of a:
1. Maxillary molar
2. Mandibular molar
3. Maxillary premolar
4. Mandibular premolar

5. The dental tissue that most closely resembles bone is:
1. Pulp
2. Dentin
3. Enamel
4. Cementum

6. Which of the following may cause food impaction or retention?
A. Defective contact points
B. Unrestored carious lesions
C. Aberrant swallowing patterns
D. Discrepancies in marginal ridge height
1. (a), (b) and (c)
2. (a), (b), and (d)
3. (a), (c) and (d)
4. (a) and (d) only
5. (b) and (c) only
6. (c) and (d) only

7. When examining permanent teeth in intercuspal position, which of the following relations are noted for a patient with normal occlusion?
A. Each tooth occludes with two opposing teeth
B. The maxillary arch is larger than the mandibular arch, producing acceptable horizontal overlap
C. Mandibular posterior teeth are anterior to maxillary posterior teeth
D. Interproximal spaces in maxillary and mandibular arches coincide only at midline

1. (a), (b) and (c)
2. (a), (b) and (d)
3. (b), (c) and (d)
4. (c) and (d) only
5. All of the above

8. The effects of acid on enamel are governed by the:

A. pH of plaque
B. Buffering capacity of saliva
C. Susceptibility of the tooth surface
D. Concentration of calcium and phosphorus in plaque

1. (a) and (b) only
2. (a), (b) and (c)
3. (a), (c) and (d)
4. (b) and (c) only
5. (b), (c) and (d)
6. All of the above

Section 6

1. The gingiva of the facial aspect of maxillary anterior teeth of an 11-year-old patient is red, edematous and bleeds easily. The affected area is widest in the midline and tapers laterally. The remaining gingiva is normal. This condition is most likely due to:

1. Occlusal trauma
2. Mouth breathing
3. Puberty hyperplasia
4. Vitamin C deficiency
5. Allergy to a dentrifice
6. Self-inflicted gingival trauma

2. Which premolar often has three cusps?

1. Maxillary first
2. Maxillary second
3. Mandibular first
4. Mandibular second

3. Application of excessive heat to a tooth results in pain because:

1. All stimuli to the pulp result in a pain sensation

2. Excessive stimulation of a heat receptor always results in pain
3. Heat receptors in the pulp have a low threshold to pain
4. Blood vessels of the pulp expand and cause strangulation of the tissue

4. A hard, dark brown or black spot on the clinical crown of a tooth of a 56-year-old patient is most likely

1. Arrested caries
2. Melanin deposition in tooth structure
3. Mercury from amalgam placement staining the tooth
4. Hemorrhage and subsequent degradation of the blood clot

5. Which of the following types of ridges is unique feature of a permanent maxillary molars?

1. Cuspal
2. Oblique
3. Transverse
4. Triangular

6. Lateral (accessory) pulp canals extend:

1. Vertically toward the cementum
2. Between two pulp canals, as a bridge
3. From the chamber, parallel to another canal
4. From pulp tissue to the periodontal ligament

7. Which of the following relations are found in a patient with normal occlusion?

A. Each tooth occludes with two opposing teeth
B. The maxillary arch is larger than the mandibular arch, producing acceptable horizontal overlap
C. Mandibular posterior teeth are anterior to maxillary posterior teeth
D. Interproximal spaces in maxillary and mandibular arches coincide only at midline

1. (a), (b) and (c)
2. (a), (b) and (d)
3. (b), (c) and (d)
4. (c) and (d) only
5. All of the above

8. Food impaction is generally contributed by which of the following conditions?

A. Open contacts
B. Hyperplastic enamel
C. Unrestored carious lesions
D. Discrepencies in marginal ridge height
  1. (a), (b) and (c)
  2. (a), (b) and (d)
  3. (a) and (c) only
  4. (a), (c) and (d)
  5. (b), (c) and (d)

Section 7

1. A patient with maxillary incisor protrusion, and anterior openbite, crowded lower anteriors, and a high-palatal vault, most likely caused by?

A. Thumbsucking
B. Mouth breathing
C. Tongue thrushing
D. Using a pacifier
E. Nocturnal bruxism

2. A false-negative response to an electrical pulp test can be caused due to all except?

A. A tooth being immature
B. Failure to use a conductive paste
C. The operator wearing surgical gloves
D. The patients being apprehensive about the test
E. The patient being premedicated with an analgesic

3. Which of the following permanent premolars frequently lacks a transverse ridge?

A. Maxillary first
B. Maxillary second
C. Mandibular first
D. Mandibular second

Section 8

1. **The mandibular permanent second molar differs from the mandibular permanent first molar in the number of:**
   A. Cusps
   B. Roots
   C. Lingual grooves
   D. Marginal ridges

2. **The largest cusp of the maxillary permanent first molar is the:**
   A. Distobuccal
   B. Mesiobuccal
   C. Distolingual
   D. Mesiolingual

3. **The height of contour of the buccal surface of the mandibular permanent first molar is at the:**
   A. Junction of the occlusal and middle thirds
   B. Center
   C. Junction of the cervical and middle thirds

4. **The most distinguishable difference between the maxillary first and second permanent premolars is in:**
   A. The size of the crown
   B. The curvature of the facial surface
   C. The number of roots
   D. The length of the lingual cusp

5. **With the exception of the third molars, the greatest variation in occlusal anatomy is found on:**
   A. Maxillary second molars
   B. Mandibular second molars
   C. Mandibular second premolars
   D. Mandibular first premolars

6. **The permanent tooth that has the longest crown is the:**
   A. Maxillary lateral incisor
   B. Maxillary central incisor
   C. Mandibular canine
   D. Maxillary first molar

7. The anterior tooth most likely to have a bifurcated root is the permanent:

A. Maxillary canine
B. Mandibular canine
C. Maxillary central incisor
D. Mandibular lateral incisor

8. What tooth occasionally exhibits a lingual groove that extends from the enamel onto the cemental area of the root?

A. Maxillary canine
B. Maxillary third molar
C. Mandibular second premolar
D. Maxillary lateral incisor

9. The primary function of the dental pulp is to:

A. Form dentin
B. Protect the periodontium
C. Assure root-end closure
D. Prevent multiple foramina

10. Which teeth have the most variable crown shape of all permanent teeth?

A. Maxillary lateral incisors
B. Maxillary third molars
C. Mandibular lateral incisors
D. Mandibular second premolars

11. The characteristic common to all mandibular first premolars when viewed from the occlusal aspect is:

A. The middle buccal lobe makes up the majority of the tooth
B. The buccal ridge is flat
C. The marginal ridges are underdeveloped
D. The lingual cusp is large

12. The mental foramen is located closest to the:

A. Mandibular canine
B. Mandibular second premolar
C. Mandibular first molar
D. Maxillary first premolar

13. In comparison with the mandibular permanent canine, the maxillary permanent canine in the same mouth:

A. Has a shorter root
B. Is wider mesiodistally
C. Is narrower mesiodistally
D. Has a less pronounced cingulum

14. The posterior permanent tooth most likely to have a pronounced concavity on its mesial surface is the:

A. Maxillary first premolar
B. Maxillary second premolar
C. Mandibular first molar
D. Mandibular first premolar

15. The mesial contact area of a maxillary permanent lateral incisor is usually located:

A. On the incisal third of the crown
B. At the junction of the middle and incisal thirds of the crown
C. At the junction of the middle and cervical thirds of the crown
D. At the middle of the middle third

16. The permanent maxillary tooth that has the longest length of the crown is the:

A. Lateral incisor
B. Central incisor
C. Canine
D. First molar

17. The maxillary permanent first molar viewed from the occlusal has the following shape:

A. Square
B. Rectangular
C. Obtuse
D. Rhomboid

18. The hard tissue forming the largest portion of the tooth is the:

A. Enamel
B. Cementum
C. Dentin
D. Alveolus

19. Of the following dental structures, which one is found on both anterior and posterior permanent teeth?

A. Mamelons
B. Oblique ridges
C. Marginal ridges
D. Cingulum
E. Transverse ridges

20. The maxillary central incisors erupt at approximately which of the following ages?

A. 7-8 years
B. 6 years
C. 9 years
D. 5 years

21. A cingulum is normally located at the:

A. Incisal third of the lingual surface of anterior teeth
B. Middle third of the lingual surface of anterior teeth
C. Cervical third of the lingual surface of anterior teeth
D. Cervical third of the lingual surface of posterior teeth

22. The pulp horns most likely to be exposed accidentally in the preparation of a Class II cavity in the maxillary first molar are the:

A. Mesiobuccal and mesiolingual
B. Mesiolingual and distolingual
C. Distolingual and distobuccal
D. Distobuccal and mesiobuccal

23. A small enamel projection located in the cingulum area of maxillary or mandibular anterior permanent teeth is called:

A. An enamel pearl
B. A talon cusp
C. A supernumerary tooth
D. A marginal ridge

24. Lingual fossae are generally found on the:

A. Lingual surface of mandibular premolars
B. Lingual surface of maxillary premolars
C. Lingual surface of anterior teeth
D. Lingual surface of mandibular molars

25. A small nodule of enamel with a tiny core of dentin, found most frequently in the furcation area of maxillary molars is called:

A. A talon cusp
B. A tubercle
C. Accessory ridges
D. An enamel pearl

Answer Key to MCQs in Sections 1–8

Section 1

1	2	2	4	3	3	4	5
5	4	6	1	7	4	8	1
9	2	10	7	11	3	12	1
13	2	14	5	15	5	16	3

Section 2

1	3	2	3	3	1	4	1
5	5						

Section 3

1	4	2	3	3	4

Section 4

1	1	2	1	3	2	4	5
5	1	6	3	7	5	8	2
9	2	10	3				

Section 5

1	3	2	2	3	2	4	1
5	4	6	2	7	3	8. Not Scored	

Section 6

1	2	2	4	3	1	4	1
5	2	6	4	7	3	8	4

Section 7

1. (A) The pressure of the thumb against the palate and maxillary teeth during the growth and development of the teeth and oral cavity can cause anterior open bite and overjet, labial flare of the maxillary anterior teeth, and high palatal vault.
2. (D) A patient who is apprehensive about a pulp test might respond to the electric stimulus when no actual sensation is felt, which can result in a false-positive response.
3. (B) The mandibular second premolar tooth has either two or three cusps. The two-cusp type (43 percent) has a transverse ridge, while the three-cusp type (54 percent) does not.

Section 8

1	A	2	D	3	C	4	C
5	C	6	C	7	B	8	D
9	A	10	B	11	A	12	B
13	B	14	A	15	B	16	B
17	D	18	C	19	C	20	A
21	C	22	A	23	B	24	C
25	D						

13

Microbiology

Prokaryotes = include bacteria, blue green algae

Eukaryotes = include fungi, algae, slime moulds, protozoa

Difference between pro- and eukaryotes =

- Prokaryotes have one, **circular chromosome;** eukaryotes- have > 1, linear chromosome
- In CW, muramic acid and diaminopimelic acid are present in prokaryotes, but absent in eukaryotes.
- Nuclear memb, nucleolus, deoxyribonucleoprotein, mitochondria, golgi, lysosome, ER, sterols are absent in prokaryotes.
- Bacteria are prokaryotes which do not contain CHLOROPHYLL.

Limit of resolution with unaided eye is = 200 microns

In **phase contrast microscopy** = phase differences are converted in differences of light, so light and dark contrast are produced in the image.

Dark field microscope = here, reflected light is used instead of transmitted light, e.g. spirochetes detection

With visible light = limit of resolution is 300 nm.

In order to be seen and resolved = an object should have a size of approx half the wavelength of the light used.

Interference microscope = also enables the quantitative measurements of chemical constituents of the cells.

Electron microscope = resolving power is 0.1 nm. In it, gas molecules scatter the electrons, so the object should **be examined in vacuum;** only dead and dried objects should be examined.

STAINING

1. Supravital = ie during which the cell is killed.
2. Vital/intra vital = ie cell retain its viability
3. Bacteria have an affinity for basic dyes due to acidic nature of their protoplasm
4. Simple stains = provide color contrast, but impart same color to the bacteria
5. Negative stains = background is colored by dyes; unstained bacteria stand out in contrast, e.g. spirochetes, bacterial capsule.
6. Impregnation method = very thin cells and structures can be seen by impregnation with Ag, e.g. spirochetes
7. Differential stains = give different color to different bacteria/ bacterial structures, e.g. Gram stain, acid fast stains
8. G + = resist discolorisation, retain primary color , VIOLET; have more acidic protoplasm so retain basic dyes.
9. G — = get discolorisation; seen RED colored.
10. Acid fast stains = TB resists discolorisation after staining with aniline dyes, AFB retains RED color; acid fastness is due to high contents of lipids, Fatty acids, alcohols, esp **mycolic acid**

SHAPE

➤ COCCI	➤ Spherical/oval	➤ Diplococcus	➤ In pairs
➤ BACILLI	➤ rod shaped	➤ streptococcus	➤ in chains
➤ VIBRIOS	➤ comma-shaped	➤ tetrads	➤ in fours
➤ SPRILLA	➤ rigid, spiral form	➤ sarcina	➤ in eights
➤ SPIROCHETES	➤ flexuous, spiral form	➤ staphylococcus	➤ grape like clusters

- **actinomycetes** = branching, filamentous bacteria; resemble **sun-ray**; rigid cell wall is present.
- **Mycoplasmas** = bacteria are cell wall **deficient,** when cell wall synthesis is deficient- the bacteria loose their distinctive form. Such cells are ka **protoplast, spheroplast** or L-form.
- Bacilli arranged at angles/**Chinese – letter form** = coryne-bacterium. The arrangement is due to **plane of binary fission.**

MORPHOLOGY OF BACTERIA

- Outer layer/cell envelope = a rigid cell wall + cytoplasmic/plasma membrane
- Flagella = for locomotion
- Fimbriae = **for adhesion**
- Cell wall = gives shape, rigidity, ductility. It can be seen by *plasmolysis* ie when bacterium is placed in hypertonic solution – the cytoplasm looses water and shrinks; but CW retains original shape/ size. It is ka *Bacterial Ghost.*
- CW is formed of N- acetyl glucosamine and N – acetyl muramic acid. (Naga and Nama)
- Endotoxic activity and O-Antigen specificity of G (-) bacteria is due to presence of lipopolysaccharides, aka **Bovine Ag.**
- *Lysozyme* = splits CW mucopolypeptide linkages. In G + bacteria, it forms PROTOPLAST and in G (-) bact, it forms SPHEROPLAST.
- Cytoplasmic membrane = is semipermeable; due to specific enzymes ie permeases; sterols are absent except in mycoplasma.
- Cytoplasm = differs from prokaryotes; it does not have internal mobility ie **protoplasmic streaming**.
- Ribosomes = protein synthesis occurs; form **polysomes** when get integrated in linear strands with mRNA.
- **Mesosomes / chondroids** = are invaginations of plasma membrane into cytoplasm. More prominent in G + bacteria, are PRINCIPAL SITES OF RESPIRATORY ENZYMES. And are equivalent to mitochondria of eukaryotes. Help to coordinate the nuclear and cytoplasmic division during binary fission.
- **Intra cytoplasmic inclusions** = e.g. volutin granules / **Babe – Ernst granules** are characteristic of **Diphtheria bacillus.**
- Nucleus = no nuclear membrane or nucleolus; DNA is double stranded and CIRCULAR; chromosome is haploid and replicate by simple fission
- **Plasmids / episomes** = *extranuclear* genetic material of DNA;

- **Capsule swelling / Quellung reaction** = seen in **Pneumococci**
- Capsule = protects bacteria from lytic enzymes; contribute to virulence; protects from phagocytosis; is antigenic.
- **Flagella** = are organs of locomotion; made of FLAGELLIN

➢ **Peritrichous**	➢ Flagella all around the cell, e.g. typhoid bacilli
➢ **Monotrichous**	➢ Flagella at single end / pole, e.g. cholera vibrio
➢ **Lophotrichous**	➢ Flagella in tufts, e.g. spirilla
➢ **Amphitrichous**	➢ Flagella at both ends

- **Fimbriae** = in G (-) bacilli; aka pili; contain protein **pilin;** are organ of adhesion; can be detected by HAEMAGGLUTINATION; by electron microscope.
- **Sex pilus** = found in **male bacteria;** form conjugation tube.
- Spores = esp of genera clostridium and bacillus; not a method of reproduction but RESTING phase; are *endospores* as they are formed inside the cell; position may be terminal, subterminal and central. Get destroyed at 120° C for 15 min in autoclave, at 15 psi.
- **GROWTH OF BACTERIA** = by **binary fission;** grow by geometric progression.

Bacterial growth curve = 4 stages ie

- **Lag phase** = no increase in the no. but increase in size; it is the **time required for adaptation** to new atmosphere. **Cell size is maximum** in this stage.
- **Log phase / exponential phase** = cell divides; their **no. increases** exponentially; size decreases;
- **Stationary phase** = cell division comes to a halt due to depletion of nutrients; viable **cell count remains constant; SPORULATION** occurs; exotoxins and antibiotics are produced in it.
- **Phase of decline** = **no. decrease** due to death of cells.

- NUTRITION = water, carbon, nitrogen and inorganic salts are required.
- **Phototrophs** = bacteria which derive their energy from sunlight.
- **Chemotrophs** = bacteria which derive their energy from chemical reactions.
- **Autotrophs** = bacteria which can synthesise all their organic compounds, are not of medical importance.
- **Heterotrophs** = bacteria which can not synthesise their own metabolites & depend on preformed organic compounds.
- **Aerobic** = require oxygen for growth.
- **Obligate aerobes** = grow in presence of oxygen only, e.g. cholera vibrio.
- **Facultative anaerobes** = which are ordinarily aerobic, but can grow also in absence of oxygen.; mostly of MEDICAL IMPORTANCE.
- **ANAEROBIC** = grow in absence of oxygen; die in presence of oxygen.
- **Microaerophilic** = grow best in p.o low oxygen tension. Enzyme **catalase** is present in most aerobes but not in anaerobes. It splits H_2O_2 to H_2O and nascent O.

- Oxidative phosphorylation gives energy ie ADP → to ATP.

TEMPERATURE

- Optimum temperature = at which best growth occurs; is 37° C; most of the pathogenic bacteria,

- **mesophilic** = at 25 – 40° C; *best growth;* all parasites of warm blooded animals.
- **Psychrophilic** = best grow at temperature < 20° C; eg saprophytes.
- **Thermophilic** = grow best at high temperature; 55 – 80° C.

- Moist heat = causes coagulation and denaturation of proteins; is more lethal.

- Dry heat = causes oxidation and charring.
- Drying is lethal to bacteria; but spores are resistant.
- Thermal death point = ie lowest temperature required to kill a bacterium in a given time under standard conditions.
- Drying in vacuum / freeze drying / lyophilisation = helps preserve the bacteria, virus etc.
- Majority of pathogenic bacteria grow at 7.2 –7.6 pH.
- Strong solutions of acid / alkali, e.g. 5 % HCl, or NaOH readily kill bacteria, but TB are resistant.
- Grow well in dark, but sensitive to UV light.
- **Plasmolysis** = if bacteria placed in hypertonic solution, water of the cell goes out and shrinkage occurs.
- **Plasmoptysis** = in hypotonic solution – bacteria swell and ruptured.

STERILIZATION

Sterilization = is the process that completely destroys all forms of microbial life including spores.

Disinfection = here, liquid chemicals are used to destroy pathogenic bacteria on INANIMATE surfaces.

Antisepsis = here, liquid chemicals are used to destroy pathogenic bacteria **on animate objects**;

Sanitization = here, a good cleaning process or boiling is done to destroy bacteria.

Sepsis = is the breakdown of living tissues by the action of bacteria and is usually accompanied by inflammation.

Asepsis = is the avoidance of sepsis.

Sterility = the freedom from viable forms of microorganism.

Bactericidal = ie which are able to kill the bacteria;

Bacteriostatic = prevent the multiplication of bacteria and they may remain alive.

Pathogens = ie those bacteria capable of producing disease.

Non-pathogens = are harmless and have no connection with disease.

Benzalkonium chloride (the quarternary ammonium compounds) are used for sanitisation and house keeping cleaning.

Sunlight = mainly **UV rays** are germicidal.

Drying = spores are unaffected by drying.

Hot air oven	160 C/ 1 hr; 180 C / 20 min.	
Autoclave	121 C / 15 – 20 min./15 psi	Perfect method
Boiling water bath	100 C / 10 – 20 min	No spore destroyed
Pasteurization of milk and butter	**Holder method** = 63 C / 30 min. **Flash method** = 72 C / 20 sec.	
Tyndallization or intermittent sterilization	100 C / 20 min for 3 consecutive days.	
Asbestos / Seitz filters		
Mambrane filters	Made of cellulose esters/ aka millepore filters	
Non-ionising radiations	UV; 250 – 260 nm; interferes with DNA replication; spores are highly resistant;	May cause retinal detachment
Ionising radiations/aka cold sterilisation	X-rays/gamma-/ cosmic rays; spores are more resistant; used in large commercial	

	plant **for mass sterilization;**	
Phenols; 1 %; eg in Dettol (chloroxylenol)	Cause cell membrane damage so releasing cell contents and causing cell lysis.	Little active vs spores
Alcohol	Denatures the bacterial proteins	
Cationic surface active agents	Act on the PO4 group of cell membrane. And enter in the cells; membrane looses its permeability; cell proteins are denatured;	

Heat = most reliable; the time required for sterilization is inversely proportional to the temperature of exposure.

Bacterial spores can be killed **by dry heat** at 160° C/1 hr ; or 180° C/20 min.

Dry heat is less effective than moist heat.

Moist heat causes **denaturation and coagulation of** bacterial proteins.

Sterilization check = by growing the spores of the bacterium BACILLUS STEARO-THERMOPHILUS and / or spores of bacillus subtilis subsp. Niger.

House hold utensils and patients clothing may be disinfected = in water at 70 – 80° C for several minutes.

Low temperature steam – **formaldehyde** sterilization = ie disinfection of objects at 75° C with formaldehyde vapors at subatmospheric pressure.

Irritant residues of HCHO vapors can be removed by = exposure of the disinfected articles to AMMONIA VAPORS.

Alcohol = should be used at 60 – 70 % conc. as water is essential for antimicrobial activity.

Dyes = more active vs G (+) than G (—) bacteria; they interfere with the synthesis of the peptidoglycan component of the cell wall.

Ethylene oxide gas = highly effective vs spores and TB bacteria; its explosive nature can be controlled by using a mixture of 10 % ethylene oxide gas with **carbon dioxide gas.** It has alkylating action on proteins and inhibition of enzymatic activity.

Surface active agents = reduce the surface tension; eg cationic compounds. They lead to **loss of membrane semipermeability** and leakage from the cell ; denatures proteins; eg cetrimide/ cetavalon.

Disinfection of operation theater = fumigation by formaldehyde solution in water placed in an electric boiler for 24 hrs; **residual formaldehyde is removed with ammonia gas.**

Moist heat sterilization = Autoclave

CULTURE MEDIA

Simple media / basal media	Eg nutrient broth, which has peptone + meat extract + NaCl + H_2O
Nutrient agar	2 % agar + nutrient broth
Enriched media	Blood/ serum / egg added to basal medium
Enrichment media	ie substance added to media to **allow growth of wanted bacteria,** e.g. tetrathionate broth for typhoid – paratyphoid bacilli
Indicator media	Indicator which change color when bacteria grow
Differential media	ie they bring out differing characteristic of bacteria and thus help to distinguish between them, e.g. MacConkey's media shows lactose fermenters as pink colonies, while non- lactose fermenters as colorless.
Transport media	Eg for gonococci., Stuart's media
Anaerobe media	Eg Robertson's cooked meat (RCM) media
McIntosh and Filde's jar	For anaerobic culture

Selective media

1. Borrelia	Noguchi's medium
2. Clostridia	Robertson's cooked meat medium/ RCM
3. Corynebacterium	Loeffler's medium / LSS
4. Fungi	Sabouraud's agar
5. Staphylococci	8 – 10 % NaCl – tellurite medium in solid broth
6. TB bacillus	Lowenstein–Jansen medium / LJ
7. Transport of streptococci	Pikes medium

BACTERIAL GENETICS

1. DNA on **transcription** forms RNA; RNA on **translation** forms polypeptide.
2. **Codon** = has sequence of 3 bases ie **triplet**. It is specific and degenerate.
3. **Non- sense codons** = 3 ie UAA, UGA, UAG; act as **stop codons** terminating the synthesis of polypeptides.
4. **Cistron / gene** = segment of DNA carrying codons for a particular polypeptide.
5. Bacterial DNA = double stranded; **circular.**
6. **Introns** = several stretches of DNA which do not appear to function as codons occur between the coding sequences of genes; are non-coding.
7. **Exons** = are the stretches of coding / coded genes.
8. **Extrachromosomal genetic material** in bacteria = (1) **Plasmids** = consist of DNA situated in cytoplasm in free state and reproduce autonomically. (2) **Episomes** = exist as either autonomously in the cytoplasm or in the integrated state, attached to bacterial chromosome. They give rise to drug – resistance, toxigenicity, maleness. After conjugation, the recipient acquires the plasmid and becomes male; thus **maleness is infectious;** such plasmids

are ka TRANSMISSIBLE PLASMIDS., e.g. drug – resistance factor in enterobacteria.

9. **Transduction** = transfer of DNA from one bacteria to other by BACTERIOPHAGE , which are viruses parasiting the bacteria. Episomes and plasmids may also be transferred,; can be used to treat some inborn errors of metabolism. It is the form of bacterial gene transfer which is **least susceptible to DNA ase** and does not require cell to cell contact ie is thro the bacteriophages.
10. **Transformation** = is the transfer of genetic material thro the agency of free DNA. Eg in **pneumococci**, bacillus species, H. influenzae.
11. **Lysogenic conversion** = in **diphtheria bacilli.** 1. **Virulent** / lytic cycle = ie large no. of progeny phases are built up in the host bacterium, which ruptures to release them. 2. **Temperate** / non-lytic cycle = host bact remains unharmed, the phage DNA becomes integrated with the bact chromosome as **prophage,** which multiplies synchronously with host DNA and is transferred to daughter cells. It is ka lysogeny. Bacteria harbouring them are ka lysogenic. Eg in **diphtheria bacilli**
12. **Conjugation** = male bacteria mates with female bacteria, which then gets converted in male. Plasmid in male help in forming sex – pilus / conjugation tube, it is ka sex factor / **fertility factor.**
13. F – factor is a transfer factor for synthesis of sex pilus but is devoid of other genetic markers, e.g. drug resistance.
14. **Col factor/ colcinogenic** = some strains of coliform bacteria produce COLICINS, i.e. antibiotic substance which are selectively and specifically lethal to enterobacteria. Colicin production is determined by a plasmid ka col factor.
15. RTF, i.e. resistance transfer factor = is a plasmid having 2 components ie R = RTF + r – factor
16. RTF = is responsible for conjugational transfer.
17. **R –factor** = resistance determinant = for each of the several drug. Resistance to >= 8 drugs can be transferred at a time. It is ka **transferrable drug resistance**, and seen in enterobacteria, vibrio, pseudomonas.

18. **Mutational drug resistance** = involves **one drug** resistance at a time.
19. **Transposons** = those DNA segments which can move around b/w chromosomal and extra chromosomal DNA molecules within a cell. This mode of genetic transfer is ka **transposition.**

INFECTIONS

SAPROPHYTES	Free living microbes which subsist on dead/ decaying organic matter. Found in soil and water, play an imp **role in degradation of organic material**, not capable of multiplying on living tissues.
PARASITES	➢ Microbes which can multiply in hosts. ➢ **Pathogens** = ie produce disease ➢ **Commensals** = live in complete harmony with host ➢ **Facultative pathogens** = produce disease if host resistance decreases.
PRIMARY INFECTION	Initial infection with a parasite in a host.
REINFECTION	Subsequent infection by **same parasite** in a host
SECONDARY INFECTION	Infection by a **new parasite** in a host whose resistance has been lowered by some primary infection
CROSS INFECTION	If in a patient already having an infection, another infection sets in from some other host.
NOSOCOMIAL INFECTION	Cross infection occurring **in an hospital.**
IATROGENIC INFECTION	Infection induced by a doctor

INFECTIONS (*Contd.*)

ENDOGENOUS INFECTION	If source of infection is host's own body
EXOGENOUS INFECTION	If source of infection is from external source
INAPPARENT/ SUBCLINICAL INFECTION	ie when clinical effects are not apparent
ATYPICAL INFECTION	In which, typical clinical effects are not present
LATENT INFECTION	Some parasites remain in dormant stage, but proliferate and produce clinical disease when host resistance is decreased.
CARRIER	ie a person who harbours the pathogenic microorganisms without suffering from any ill effects from it.
HEALTHY CARRIER	Who harbours a pathogen but **has never suffered from the disease** caused by that pathogen
CONVALESCENT CARRIER	Who has **recovered from the disease** but continues to harbour the pathogen in the body
TEMPORARY CARRIER STAGE	For < 6 months
CHRONIC CARRIER STAGE	For many years
CONTACT CARRIER	Person who acquires the pathogen from a patient
PARADOXICAL CARRIER	Who acquires pathogen from another carrier

INFECTIONS (*Contd.*)

RESERVOIR HOST	*Animals* serving as to maintain the parasite in nature and act as reservoir of human infection
ZOONOSES	Disease transmitted **from animals to man**, e.g. plague, rabies, hydatid, etc.
ANTHROPOZOO-NOSES	Disease spreading **from vertebrates** and animals to man.
EPIZOOTIC	
ANTHROPOID BORNE DISEASE	Blood sucking *insects* may transmit pathogens to man, e.g. mosquitos, ticks, flies etc. act as vectors.
MECHANICAL VECTORS	ie infection transmitted by vectors *without any life cycle* of pathogen in the vector
BIOLOGICAL VECTOR	ie when pathogen passes a part of its development cycle in the vector, e.g. anopheles mosquito in malaria.
EXTRINSIC INCUBATION PERIOD	ie the time required for the biological vector to become infective beginning from the time of entry of pathogen into it.
BY DIRECT CONTACT	Disease are said to be contagious
INFECTIOUS DISEASE	ie disease caused by all other means
FOMITES	Are **inanimate objects** causing indirect contact and infection transmission., e.g. trachoma by towels of the patient
INOCULATION	ie pathogens *directly deposited* in host tissue, e.g. rabies, tetanus, HIV, HBV etc.
INHALATION	Infection by droplet nuclei, e.g. TB

INFECTIONS (Contd.)

VERTICAL TRANSMISSION	ie infection from mother to fetus. Eg rubella, congenital syphilis
HORIZONTAL TRANSMISSION	Infection from one person to another
PATHOGENICITY	Ability of a microbial species to produce disease
VIRULENCE	Is the same (as above) property in a strain of microorganism.
EXALTATION	Enhancement of virulence
ATTENUATION	Reduction of virulence
COMMUNI-CABILITY	Ability of a parasite to spread from one host to another
BACTERAEMIA	Circulation of bacteria in blood
SEPTICAEMIA	Bacteria circulate and multiply in blood, form toxic products, cause high swinging type of fever.
PYAEMIA	Pyogenic bacteria produce septicemia with multiple abscesses in internal organs
ENDEMIC DISEASE	Disease which is **constantly present** in a particular area
EPIDEMIC	One which **spreads very rapidly** involving many persons in an area at the same time.
PANDEMIC	Is an epidemic which spreads thro many areas of the **world,** involving very large no. of persons within a short period.
PROSDEMIC	Creeping / smouldering epidemic which spreads **very slowly** by person to person contact.

DIFFERENCE B/W EXOTOXINS and ENDOTOXINS

EXOTOXINS	ENDOTOXINS
Protein in nature	Protein – polysaccharides – lipid
Heat labile	Stable
Active secretion from cell	Form **part of cell wall;** toxicity depends on lipid content
Active in *very minute doses*	Large doses required
Highly **antigenic**	Weak
Action can be neutralised by specific antibodies	No
Can be **toxoided**	No
Mainly produced by G + bacteria, but some G – bact also produce	Only by G -
Diffuse in surrounding media	Do not.

Bacterial products may contribute to virulence of bacteria by inhibiting mechanism of host resistance, for example:

1. Coagulase produced by staphylococci = **prevents phagocytosis** by forming a fibrin barrier around bacteria and walling the lesion.
2. Fibrinolysin = **helps spread of infections** by breaking down the fibrin barrier in the tissues.
3. Hyaluronidase = split hyaluronic acid in connective tissues and helps spreading of infections along the tissue spaces.
4. Leucocidin = damage PMN cells.
5. Hemolysins = damage RBCs.
6. Capsulated bacteria = are not readily phagocytosed.

IMMUNITY

- Is the resistance of host towards the injury caused by microorganisms and their products.

- **Types** = I. innate immunity = specific; nonspecific.
  II. Acquired immunity =
  a. active = natural ; artificial
  b. passive = natural ; artificial.
- **Innate / native immunity** = is the resistance to infections which an individual possesses by his genetic and constitutional make – up. It does not depend on prior contact with microorganisms and immunisation. It is **obtained as a birth right**.
- **Mechanism of innate I** =

1. Intact skin / epithelial surface act as barrier to invasion. Skin has antibacterial activity due to **high salt in sweat**.
2. Saliva, nasal and respiratory secretions
3. Phagocytes
4. Acidic pH of gastric juices.
5. Tears contain lysozymes. Lysozymes are found in all tissue fluids and secretions **except** CSF, sweat, urine.
6. In blood = complements have bactericidal activity; **properdine** present in normal serum cause lysis of G (-) bacteria.
7. Interferones = act vs viruses.

- **Acquired immunity** = is the resistance that an individual acquires during life. 2 types —

Active	Passive
Develops due to antigenic stimulus	Resistance transmitted in ready made mode. Eg by vaccines. No Agic stimulus
Antibodies produced by patient's immune system	Preformed Abs are introduced
Sets in after a **latent period**	**Immediate effect**
Long lasting, More effective and better.	Transient, less effective, inferior

Active	**Passive**
Secondary response is seen ie in actively immunised patient vs some Ag, if the same Ag is encountered again, the response is fast and abundant.	No sec. Response. **Immune elimination** ie when a foreign Ag is administered second time, it is eliminated more rapidly than initially. So it limits the usefulness of repeated passive immunisation.
Immunologic memory is seen	
Negative phase seen	No

Natural active immunity : results from a clinical or non-apparent infection with a parasite. Eg measles; polio; chicken pox; influenza; common cold. It is LONG –LASTING.

PREMUNITION = special type of immunity seen in **syphilis**. In it, immunity remains till original infection is active. Once the disease is cured, the patient becomes susceptible to spirochetes again.

Artificial active immunity: resistance is induced **by vaccines.**

VACCINES

1. Bacterial vaccines

a. Live = BCG for TB

b. Killed = TAB for enteric fever/typhoid.

II. Viral vaccines

a. Live = oral polio (sabin), MMR

b. **K**illed = sal**k** for polio; rabies; Hep B

III. **Bacterial products** = toxoids for diphtheria and tetanus.

IMMUNISATION SCHEDULE

AGE	VACCINE
Birth	BCG Oral polio = 1st dose Hepatitis B vaccine = 1st dose
6 weeks	DPT = 1st dose Oral polio = 2nd dose Hepatitis B vaccine = 2nd dose
Optional, 10 weeks	Hib vaccine = 1st dose DPT = 2nd dose Oral polio = 3rd dose
Optional, 14 weeks	Hib vaccine = 2nd dose DPT = 3rd dose Oral polio = 4th dose
Optional, 6 months	Hib vaccine = 3rd dose Oral polio = 5th dose Hepatitis B = 3rd dose
9 months	Measles vaccine
15 months	Hib booster
15 – 18 mos.	MMR DPT = 1st booster Oral polio = 1st booster
2 – 3 yrs	Typhoid vaccine
5 yrs	DPT = 2nd booster Oral polio = 2nd booster
6 yrs	Typhoid v.
9 yrs	Typhoid v
10 yrs	TT toxoid, Hepatitis B = booster

IMMUNISATION SCHEDULE (*Contd.*)

15 – 16 yrs	TT toxoid
Optional	Chicken pox / varicella v. Hepatitis A v =1st dose Booster dose after 6 mos = 2nd dose
BCG	Birth
Polio	0, 6, 10, 14, wk 6 mo, 15–18 mos, 5 yrs
Hep B	0, 6 wk, 6 mo, 10 yr
DPT	6 wk, 10 wk, 14 wk, 15–18 mo, 5 yr
Hib	10 wk, 14 wk, 6 mo, 15 mo
Measles	9 mo
MMR	15–18 mo
Typhoid	2–3 yrs, 6 yr, 9 yr
TT	10 yr, 15–16 yr
Chicken pox	Optional
Hep A	Optional 2 doses

Live vaccines

- Infection is initiated without causing any injury/disease.
- **Long-lasting immunity**–booster may be required.
- Eg oral (Sabin for polio), parenteral for measles

Killed vaccines

- Less immunogenic, last for **shorter period**
- Repeated administration is required.
- At least 2 doses are required = primary and booster doses
- Eg = oral (taboral for typhoid); parenteral (provides humoral Ab response, which may be improved by ADJUVANTS, e.g. Al-PO_4 adjuvant vaccine for cholera)

Natural passive immunity

- Transferred from **mother to baby (vertical)**
- Thro placenta, colostrum (IgA- rich)
- Human fetus = starts IgM production in 20 wk i.u.
- But immunologic independence occurs at 3 mos. age only
- Transport of Ab thro placenta is ACTIVE TRANSPORT
- By active immunisation of mother during pregnancy – it is possible to improve quality of passive I. in infants, e.g. TT tetanus toxoid.

Artificial passive immunity

- Resistance passively transferred to a recipient by **giving Abs.**
- By **hyperimmune sera of animals** / human etc., e.g. ATS (horse serum). It is given parenterally, i.e. s/c for prophylaxis ; and i/v for treatment.
- It provides **immediate supply** of antitoxins in recipient's blood.
- Passive immunisation is indicated for providing immediate and temporary protection in a non- immune host, when there is insufficient time for active immunity.
- Also used to suppress active immunity, e.g. in cases of transplant surgery to prevent rejection.
- Also, Rh immune globulins given to a Rh (-) mother with a Rh + baby (RHOGAM).

Combined immunisation

- Active + passive, e.g. in tetanus by ATS + TT.

Adoptive immunity = by injecting **immunologically competent lymphocytes** ka transfer factor. Eg in lapromatous leprosy.

Local immunity = to combat infection **at the site of primary entry** of pathogen. Class of **IgA** forms major component of local immunity.

- Eg in polio, active I. by killed vaccine, which acts in blood ; oral live vaccine = **acts on intestine locally** to prevent entry and multiplication of polio virus.
- Eg influenza = killed vaccine = humoral Ab response, and live viral vaccine = intranasally – local immunity.
- Secretory IgA = produced locally **by plasma cells** is present on mucosal surfaces or in secretory glands in breast milk.

Herd immunity = overall level of immunity in a community and is relevant in the control of epidemic disease. If low then epidemic may occur.

Immunity =

- ATS gives passive immunity ie antibodies injected in the body (to a patient who was never immunised).
- Non- specific immunity by BCG = is through **activation of macrophages (Bacillus Calmet Guerin).**

ANTIGENS

- Is a substance which when introduced in the body stimulates the production of an Ab or may lead to CMI or immunologic tolerance.
- **Haptens** = are the substances which are **incapable of inducing** Ab **formation** by themselves, but can react specifically with Abs, i.e. to fasten the reaction.
- **Proantigen** = are low m.wt substances which do not induce Ab formation, but cause **delayed hypersensitivity** (CMI),
- **Cryptantigen** = not available for Ag –Ab reaction, as they are not terminal.
- Antigenic determinant / **epitome** = is the **smallest unit** of antigenicity.
- **Antigenicity** = proteins / polysaccharides are more antigenic. Lipids / nucleic acids are less.

- Closely related Ags may sometimes occur in **different biological species** / class / kingdom. These are ka HETEROPHILE Ags., e.g. **Frossmann's** antigen.
- Some heterophile Ags are responsible for some diagnostic serological tests, e.g. Weil–Felix reaction for typhoid fever; Paul – Bunnel test for infectious mononucleosis.

ANTIBODIES

- Are immunoglobulins (Ig), mostly are euglobulins; Ab activity is associated with gamma – globulin fraction.
- Synthesised **by plasma cells**
- **5 classes** = Ig G,A,M,D,E as in **decreasing conc in serum**
- Ig = Fc + Fab parts ie crystallisable + Ag binding.
- Hot – spots / hypervariable regions are involved with the formation of Ag – binding sites.
- Ag combining site of the molecule is = **aminoterminus**

Abnormal Igs

- **Bence–Jones proteins** = in multiple myeloma, a plasma cell dyscrasia, coagulates at 60° C; redissolves at 80° C.
- Ig M type are produced in Waldenstrom's macroglobulinemia.
- Cryoglobulinemia

Important points

1. IgG = protects body fluids
2. IgA = protects body surfaces
3. IgM = protects blood stream
4. IgE = mediates reaginic hypersensitivity
5. IgD = role is unknown

Antibodies

Immunoglobulins : These are glycoproteins; source for preparation of human gamma globulins **is placenta.**

Ig for autoimmune reactions	IgM
Ig **maximum in saliva,** and on mucosal surface	Salivary IgA
Ig **maximum in sulcular** fluid	Ig G
Smallest Ig, **most abundant**	Ig G
Ig that **crosses placenta**	Ig G
Warm antibodies	Ig G
Blocking antibodies	IgG
Largest immunoglobulins	IgM
First Ab formed after initial exposure to Ag	IgM
Earliest antibody to be synthesised	IgM
Natural antibodies; to ABO blood group antigens	IgM
Mainly **intravascular** immunoglobulins	IgM
Cold antibodies	IgM
Reaginic antibodies (allergies)	IgE
Heat labile Ig	IgE
Ig with **minimum half life**	IgE
Ig causing atopic allergy, anaphylaxis	IgE
Immediate hypersensitivity	IgE
Ig that **protects the surface**	Ig A
Commonest Ig **deficiency**	Ig A
Prevents adhesion of bacteria to mucosa	IgA
Ig present in **milk**	IgA and IgG
By G + bacteria	Ig G
By G – bact	IgM

IgG, maternal	IgA	IgM	IgD	IgE
Maximum in serum	2nd most abundant	Heavy aka **millionaire molecule**	—	Atopic/ reaginic Ab
80 % of total	Synthesised by *plasma* cells	*Oldest* Ig class	—	Heat labile
Both extra- and intravascular	Dimer form = connected by J–chain at Fc point., found in bile also.	Mostly intra- vascular	Mostly intra- vascular	Mostly extra-, Affinity for surface of tissue cells esp *mast cells.*
Half life = 23 days	6 –8 days	5 days	3 days	2 days
Less carbohydrate	Acts vs bact. invasion in blood	—	—	Deficiency asso with IgA deficiency
Increase in chronic malaria, kala azar, myeloma	Selectively conc. On mucosal surfaces and secretions – form Ab-paste – give local I.	-Indicates recent infection b'coz of short life. -deficiency is asso. With **septicemia**	—	Increase levels in atopic, type I allergies, eg asthma, hay fever, eczema, high levels of inte- stinal parasites.
Only Ig for *placental transfer*, giving	Inhibit adherence of bacteria on	Not transferable from placent,	—	Does not cross placenta;

IgG, maternal	**IgA**	**IgM**	**IgD**	**IgE**
natural passive I	mucosal surfaces	so its presence in fetus shows infection, e.g. congeni tal- syphilis, rubella, toxoplasm-osis.		nor fix C'
Helps phagocytosis of microbes	Does not fix C', promotes phagocytosis	More effective in immune hemolysis and opsoni-sation; bactericidal	—	Mediates Prausnitz–Kustner reaction
Is late Ab	IgA2 is dominant form in secretions		Earliest Ig synth. By the fetus, 20 wks i.u	Mainly produced in the lining of resp and intestinal tracts
Present in milk	Major Ig in **colostrum**, saliva, tears		Occur on the surface of unsti-mulated B–lympho-cytes and acts as recognition receptors for Ags, also IgM	Causes anaphy-lactic type of hyper-sensitivity

IgG, maternal IgA	IgM	IgD	IgE
Passively administered suppresses homologus Abs synthesis, e.g. in isoimmunisation of women by giving anti-Rh (D) during delivery.	Isoheamagglutinins eg anti-A, anti-B, are IgM. ♦ Initial immune response is due to IgM		

AG – AB REACTIONS

- **Affinity** = intensity of attraction b/w Ag and Ab.
- **Sensitivity of test** = ability of the test to detect even very minute quantity of Ag and Ab. In highly sensitivity test, false negative results are minimal.
- **Specificity of test** = ability of test to detect reactions b/w homologous Ags and Abs only, and with no others. In highly specific test, false positive results are absent or minimal.

DIFFERENT TESTS

Ring test	CRP; Lancefield's grouping of Strept
Slide test	VDRL for syphilis
Tube test	Kahn test for syphilis
Slide agglutination test	For blood grouping; cross matching
Tube agglutination test	Widal test for typhoid; Weil – Felix test for typhus; Paul – Bunnel test for infectious mononucleosis

DIFFERENT TESTS (*Contd.*)

Coombs/antiglobulin test	For brucellosis; detecting Rh- antibodies
CFT	Wassermann's test for syphilis
Direct immunofluorescence test	For rabies
Indirect immunoflourescence test	For treponemal Ab test for syphilis;
Radioimmuno assay	Tumor marker; drugs
ELISA	HIV; Rotavirus detection

COMPLEMENT SYSTEM: are the factors present in serum which are activated by Ag – Ab reaction only.

- 9 factors = C1 to C9.
- Heat labile;
- C – binding sites are **located on Fc part** of IgM and IgG only.
- Act in 2 pathways = classical pathway; alternate / properdin pathway. They are **common after C3 activation**.
- In alternate pathway – activation of C3 does not involve C1, 4, 2 in it.

Biosynthesis of C

- C1 = intestinal epithelium
- C2, C4 = macrophages
- C5, C8 = spleen
- C3, C6, C9 = liver
- C7 = not known
- Increased levels of C4,C3,C5,C6 is seen **in acute infections**.

Biologic effects of C

- Bacteriolysis of G +; and cytolysis of G – bacteria.
- Antiviral; phagocytosis; immune adherence;

- Amplify inflammatory responses; hypersensitivity reactions, e.g.
  C2 kinins = vasoactive amines, **increase vascular permeability**
  C3a, C5a = **anaphylotoxic**, histamine releasing; chemotactic
  C567 = **chemotactic**; reactive lysis.
- Participate in cytotoxic (type II); and immune complex (type III) hypersensitivity reactions. Eg serum sickness, Arthus reaction.
- C – components decrease in serum in – SLE; rheumatoid arthritis.
- C has role in pathogenesis of = autoimmune **hemolytic anemia**; paroxysmal nocturnal hemoglobinuria, hereditary angioneurotic **oedema**.
- C 3 is activated during blood clotting by thrombin.
- Endotoxins activate alternate C pathway.
- In endotoxic shock, = there is massive C 3 fixation and platelet adherence, → platelet lysis → DIC; thrombocytopenia.
- Depletion of C protects vs Schwartzman reaction.
- C3, C4 = required for immune adherence and contribute to defence VS pathogenic microbes.

DEFICIENCY OF following Complements LEADS TO =

♦ C1 inhibitors	♦ Hereditary angioneurotic oedema, mediated by C2 kinin release. It is treated by eACA; fresh plasma
♦ Early components of classic path C142	♦ SLE and other collagen disease
♦ C3 and its regulatory proteins, C3b inactivators	♦ Severe recurrent pyogenic infections
♦ C5 – C8	♦ Bacteremia esp G – diplococci, toxoplasmosis
♦ C9	♦ No particular disease

MICROBIOLOGY

1. **Incidence** = is a function of time ie a change in experience over a particular period of time, usually one year. It is the rate of occurrence of new disease in a population during a given interval of time.
2. **Prevalence** = proportion of a population that demonstrates a particular characteristic. It is the proportion of persons affected by a disease at a specific point in time, such as determined by a cross- sectional survey.

Functions of cells

- Phagocytes = vs invasion by microorganisms.
- Microphages = are PMN leucocytes
- Macrophages = are histiocytes, fixed RE cells, monocytes.
- Macrophages of CNS = glial cells / microglial cells.
- RE cells = removal of foreign particles which enter the body.
- Neutrophils = ingest bacteria
- Plasma cells = form **antibodies**
- Mast cells = form histamine
- B- lymphocytes = form plasma cells , which form **antibodies**
- Eosinophils = increased in **allergies**; parasitic infections
- Histiocytes = secrete lipase
- Lymphocytes = neutralizes toxins; **no phagocytosis**
- Leucocytosis = occurs in acute pyogenic bacterial infections
- Histamine = by **mast cells** and **basophils**

BACTERIA (quick revision points)

- ALL cocci are gram + ve except Neisseria.
- All bacilli are gram negative except DATTA ie diphtheria; actinomycosis; tetani Cl; tuberculous bacilli; anthrax.
- Rickettesia contains enzymes of glycolysis and Kreb's cycle
- Rickettesia and virus require = living cells for growth

- Virus = are living chemicals
- **Virion** = extracellular infectious particles.
- **Rickettesia** contains both RNA and DNA, but virus contains either RNA or DNA.
- Major cariogenic property of Strept. mutans is associated with its ability to produce = GLUCOSYL TRANSFERASE ENZYME
- Strept. pneumoniae = is well known for its large polysaccharide **capsule**.
- Phycomycosis / mucormycosis = are associated with **diabetes mellitus**.
- Botulism = does not require p.o. live organism in the body to produce the disease. It causes flaccid paralysis of skeletal muscles; due to release of ENDOTOXINS.
- Histoplasma = a fungus having both
- TB and syphilis is caused by agents which produce neither endotoxins nor exotoxins.
- In histoplasmosis = organisms are characteristically **found in RE cells**.
- Bacterial exotoxins are synthesised in = ribosomes; so protein in nature
- Final H_2 – acceptor in lactic acid-fermentation by Strept. is = pyruvic acid
- Lactic acid produced by Strept. and lactobacilli in mouth is utilised by = **veillonella**, so veillonella is an ANTICARIES BACTERIA.
- Capsulated bacteria, e.g. pneumococci, are not readily phagocytosed except in p.o. OPSONINS.
- Some bacteria, e.g. brucella, lepra bacilli **resist intracellular digestion** and may actively multiply inside the phagocytes. So here, **phagocytosis may actually help in spreading the infections** in different parts of the body.

- SABE = by alpha- hemolytic Strept., i.e. Strept. viridans
- ABE = esp. by beta-hemolytic Strept.
- **Food poisoning** = by staph

- Rheumatic fever = by group A Beta – hemolytic streptococci
- Osteomyelitis = by Staph. aureus
- Fecal contaminated water is tested for = E. coli
- **Root caries** = by Actinomyces viscosus, A. naeslundii
- Intracellular mineralisation of plaque = Bacterionema matruchotii
- Cellulitis by = Strept.
- Bacteroides melaninogenicus and B. gingivalis produce collagenase, which plays part in breakdown of PDL tissues.
- Caries initiated by = Strept. mutans
- Prominent in **deep cavities** = lactobacillus
- Dominant on **smooth surface** = S. mutans
- Dominant on **P and F** = lactobacilli
- Dominant on **root caries** = actinomyces viscosus
- **Symbiont** of Strept. = veillonella
- Bacteria which lessen damaging potential of lactic acid using it as a metabolite = veillonella and Neisseria

CML is the **only leukemia with specific chromosomal marker** ie Philadelphia chromosome.

Carcinoma of prostrate gland = increased levels of serum acid P ase.

Hypersensitivity reactions

- Tuberculin reaction = cell mediated **delayed type** hypersensitivity
- Serum sickness, Arthus reaction, wheal and flare = **humoral** response.
- Contact dermatitis, tissue transplant rejection = **cell mediated** response.
- Allograft rejection is mediated by = small lymphocytes, thro a delayed hypersensitivity reaction (T - cells).

- **Polio virus** = lesions are mostly in **anterior horns of spinal cord;** where neurons are destroyed; degeneration of Nissl bodies takes place (ie chromolysis).

- **Rabies virus** = travels **along the axoplasm** towards spinal cord and brain neuronal bodies; so **spread is unilateral** and passive (@ 3 mm / hr.); in brain they multiply and **spread along the nerve trunks** to various parts of body including salivary glands, cornea, facial skin, etc. Cornea and facial skin provide a method for ante – mortem diagnosis of human rabies.
- Pathognomonic C/F of Rabies = difficulty in drinking with intense thirst; patient is able to swallow the dry solids but not liquids due to spasm of pharynx and larynx and so hydrophobia develops.
- Death occurs due to respiratory arrest.

ONCOGENIC VIRUSES

Herpes viridae, EBV	♦ Nasopharyngeal carcinoma ♦ Burkitt's lymphoma ♦ B – cell lymphoma
HSV – 2	Cervical ca.
Papova viridae	Urogenital tumor
Hepadna viridae	Primary hepatocellular ca.
Papilloma virus	Penile / vulval / cervical ca.
Retro viridae, HTLV	Adult T – cell leukemia

Mechanism of viral oncogenesis

- **Oncogenic DNA virus** = viral DNA gets incorporated in host cell genome; host cell undergoes malignant transformation; cell is not destroyed; process resembles the lysogenic conversion in bacteria.

RNA virus/ retro virus — steps are

- Viral RNA is converted in RNA : DNA hybrid under the action of enz. Reverse transcriptase (RNA directed DNA polymerase).
- Hybrid is then converted to double stranded DNA by enz DNA directed DNA polymerase. It is ka **provirus.**

- Provirus gets incorporated into host cell genome and acts as template for viral RNA synthesis and induces cell **transformation.**
- **Oncogenes** induce tumor formation.

HIV/ AIDS

- HTLV III is associated with **human T – cell leukemia**.
- HIV = **lentivirus of retro viridae family.** It is 90 – 120 nm diameter, single **stranded RNA**; reverse transcriptase enz; has lipoprotein envelop; spikes help binding to CD 4 receptors on host cells.
- Main virus antigen = P 24
- Virus infects all **cells bearing CD_4** , e.g. T4 (helper / inducer lymphocytes), B – cells ; monocytes; macrophages (Langhans cells in dermis and alveolar macrophages in lungs, microglial / glial cells in CNS).
- HIV virus is = thermolabile; ie at 56° C / for 30 min.; or 100° C for < 1 sec; it withstands LYOPHILISATION. Susceptible to common **disinfectants**, e.g. 2% glutaraldehyde; 5% formaldehyde; 3% H_2O_2 etc.
- AIDS = depression of T4 cells functions occurs; T4 cells release less amounts of IL-2, gamma – interferons, etc. which dampen the CMI.

So **major damage is on CMI.**

- Helper T-cells are = essential for optimal B-cell functions.
- **An imp feature** is = polyclonal activation of B cells leading to hypergammaglobulinemia, it may lead to TYPE 3 HYPERSENSITIVITY.
- Levels of IgG, IgA are esp increased; IgM also in children.
- T4 cells decrease in no. and **T4 – T8 cells ratio is REVERSED.**
- C/ F = Pneumonia in AIDS is due to esp. **P. carinii.** Kaposi's sarcoma; important intestinal pathogen is CRYPTOSPORIDIUM.
- HIV can *cross blood – brain barrier*
- Virus is mostly in lymphocytes, in body fluids.

- Infections is mainly due to transfer of infected cells rather than the pure virus.
- Diagnostic tests = ELISA, western blot test.

HEPATITIS

Type A hepatitis = aka **infectious hepatitis**

- Infection spreads by faeco-oral route.
- Incubation period = 2 – 6 weeks.
- No transplacental transfer of virus.
- Most common cause of acute hepatitis in children.
- It is an **RNA virus (a picorna virus)**
- Virus can be inactivated by 1: 4000 formaldehyde / 37° C / 72 hrs and by 1 ppm chlorine for 30 min.
- Stands prolonged storage at 4° C.
- After development of clinical jaundice = the virus is rarely seen in faeces and blood.
- Detection of IgM antibodies in serum → implies recent infection
- Detection of IgG antibodies in serum → implies recent / remote infection
- Passive prophylaxis with human gamma – globulin is effective.

Type B hepatitis = **serum hepatitis**

- IP = 2 – 6 months
- Ag – Ab combination complexes → extrahepatic signs and symptoms
- Chronic active hepatitis = leads to **cirrhosis**
- Primary hepatocellular carcinoma can develop.
- Patient having HBS Ag for more than 6 months in blood are ka **chronic / persistent carriers** (M > F; adults > children).
- No natural animal reservoir of virus exists.
- Transmission of virus is mainly by percutaneous route, blood, kissing etc.

- Very minute amount (0.00001 ml), can cause infection.
- HBV is ka **Australia antigen** = it is HBS Ag, 22 nm in diameter.
- Double shelled spherical structure 42 nm in diameter = is a complete HBV aka **DANE particle.**
- It is **DNA virus** = double stranded DNA and a DNA – dependent DNA polymerase.
- It is classified under HEPADNA VIRUSES family.
- HBS Ag = is ka AUSTRALIA Ag
- HBC Ag = is ka CORE Ag.
- HBE Ag = is associated with core of virus and also with **infectivity** of carrier blood.
- HB carriers = A) **proper carriers** = ie have Hbe Ag = show early stage of carrier state; *very highly infectious;* have high titers of HbsAg; and DNA polymerase; HBV may be present.
- **Simple carriers** = has no Hbe Ag'; low levels of HBs Ag; HBV and DNA polymerase are absent. It represents later stages of carrier state.
- **Immune response** = **Ab to HBS Ag** is associated with resistance to infection;
- Ab to HBc Ag is not protective but is related to the amount and duration of replication of virus.
- Highest titres of anti-HBc are present in persistent HBs Ag carriers;
- Ab to HBe Ag is measured by leucocyte migration inhibition and development during acute phase of illness and disappears soon after recovery.
- Hepatitis B vaccine is a **recombinant vaccine** which consist of HbsAg.

Interpretation of hepatitis B serology

HbsAg, surface Ag	Virus present – infective risk
HbsAb; anti HbsAg	**Immunity** associated with clinical recovery; or previous immunization

Interpretation of hepatitis B serology

HbeAg; e antigen	**High risk infectivity**
HbeAb; anti HbeAg	Resolution of active inflammation; No special high risk infection
HbcAb, anti HBc Ag	Past or present infection
Anti HBc IgM	**Best indicator** of acute infection
Anti – HDV IgM	Indicates **recent infection**

HBs Ag	Is earliest and **specific marker** of infection;
HBc Ag	Not seen in serum of patients but can be seen in **liver cells** by immuno-fluorescence; Ab to it appears in **preicteric phase.**
Hbe Ag	Correlates with the number of viral particles and degree of infectivity of carrier sera. Sera containing it are HIGHLY INFECTIOUS; is an adverse prognostic sign.
Delta agents	Is a defective virus which needs HBV as a helper for replication, has low m. wt. RNA.
Passive immunisation	Given after an acute exposure to HB infection. Human serum Ig is given. Anti-hepatitis B immunoglobulin is preferred.
Active immunisation	With heat-inactivated human carrier plasma. 3 doses of 1 ml given I/M = at 0, 1, 6 months interval, followed by booster dose at 5 yrs.

Difference b/w type A and type B hepatitis

Properties	Type A	Type B
IP	2 – 6 wks	2 – 6 months
Onset	Acute	Slow

Difference b/w type A and type B hepatitis

Age	Children	All ages
Australia Ag	—	+
Increased IgM	+	—
Mode of infection	Oral	Parenteral
Virus size	27 nm	42 nm
Nucleic acid	RNA	DNA
Carriers	—	+
Virus in feces	+	—

NORMAL FLORA OF THE BODY

Skin = Staph, Strept. viridans; Str faecalis; Candida albicans; Mycobacterium.

Hair = Staph aureus

Mouth

- Of infant is not sterile at birth; but contains same type of bacteria as in mother's vagina.
- After 2 – 5 days = get replaced by bacteria present in mouth of the mother.
- Within 12 hrs = **alpha hemolytic Strept.** become dominant organism of oropharynx and remain so for the life.

Intestine

- In breast fed children = lactobacilli 99 % (L. bifidus)
- In bottle fed children = L. acidophilus
- In normal adult = stomach is sterile due to low pH.

No. of bacteria increase progressively beyond the duodenum to the colon; they are mostly anaerobes.

In blood = commensals may enter blood and tissues, but get quickly eliminated by normal defense mechanism of the body.

Breast milk = mostly staph epidermidis

Botryomycosis = caused by Staph. aureus

Hospital infections

- Wound infections = abscess etc by Staph. epidermidis; Strept pyogenes; Staph; Clostridia etc.
- HBV is the most imp virus causing the infections
- Pseudomonas aeruginosa = mimp cause of infection in **burns**;
- UTI = E. coli; proteus; Ps. aeruginosa; etc.
- Resp. infections = multiple drug resistant Staph aureus and G (-) bacilli;
- Bacteriemia / septicaemia = Staph epidermidis commonly in patients with **artificial heart valves**, and endocarditis.

Shape of the organisms

1. Bullet	rabies virus
2. Drumstick	Cl. tetani
3. Half moon	meningococci
4. Kidney	gonococci
5. Lanceolate	diplococci/pneumococci
6. Safety pin	plague
7. Spindle	Cl. welchi

Bacterial arrangements

• Anthrax	chains / bamboo stick appearance
• Diphtheria	Chinese letter pattern
• Enterococci	pairs
• Leprosy bacilli	cigar bundle appearance
• Meningo/gonococci	pairs mainly intracellular
• Pneumococci	pairs
• Staphylococci	bunches / irregular
• Streptococci	chains

Viral Inclusion bodies

Intracytoplasmic

1. Rabies	Negri bodies
2. Small pox	Gaurnier bodies
3. Molluscum contagiosum	Henderson–Peterson bodies

Intra nuclear bodies

• Cowdry type A	herpes virus / Lipschultz inclusion
• Cowdry type A	yellow fever / Torres bodies
• Cowdry type B	adeno virus and polio virus

Both intranuclear and intracytoplasmic

- Measles virus

14

MCQs in Microbiology and Pathology

Part I

1. **Which of the following characteristics is the most reliable indicator of prognosis of malignant tumors?**
   A. Size of tumor
   B. The degree of differentiation
   C. The degree of localization
   D. Abnormal mitoses

2. **Humans may acquire *Toxoplasma gondii* by:**
   A. Airborne conidia
   B. Ingestion of cysts in poorly cooked meat
   C. Sustaining a dog bite
   D. Swimming in contaminated water

3. **Which type of cancer listed below originates in the middle layer of the epidermis and is the most common type of oral cancer?**
   A. Basal cell carcinoma
   B. Malignant melanoma
   C. Squamous cell carcinoma
   D. Kaposi's sarcoma

4. Various species of the following bacteria produce the enzyme hyaluronidase, except:
   A. Streptococcus
   B. Clostridium
   C. Staphylococcus
   D. Neisseria

5. Quaternary ammonium compounds, which are widely used for skin antisepsis, are classified as:
   A. Nonionic detergents
   B. Anionic detergents
   C. Cationic detergents
   D. None of the above

6. All of the following are prokaryotic cells, except:
   A. Bacteria
   B. Chlamydia
   C. Fungi
   D. Mycoplasmas
   E. Rickettsia

7. Capsules play important roles in all of the following diseases, except:
   A. Haemophilus meningitis
   B. Cryptococcoses
   C. Gonorrhea
   D. Pneumococcal pneumonia
   E. Meningococcemia

8. Bacterial vaccines are composed of:
   A. Capsular polysaccharides
   B. Inactivated protein exotoxins (toxoids)
   C. Killed bacteria
   D. Live attenuated bacteria
   E. All of the above

9. The enzymes superoxide dismutase and catalase are not present in:
   A. Obligate aerobes
   B. Facultative anaerobes

C. Obligate anaerobes
D. All of the above

10. The Hepatitis A virus, Poliovirus, and Rotavirus have which portal of entry listed below?
A. Respiratory tract
B. Gastrointestinal tract
C. Skin
D. Genital tract
E. Blood

11. Which of the following are respiratory enzymes capable of undergoing alternate reduction and oxidation?
A. Pyrimidine nucleotides
B. Cytochromes
C. Reductants
D. Surfactants

12. Phlebitis can occur in any vein in the body but most often effects the:
A. Veins of the upper extremities
B. Pulmonary veins
C. Hepatic veins
D. Veins of the lower extremities

13. Which syndrome listed below is also called Trisomy 21?
A. Down syndrome
B. Edward's syndrome
C. Patau's syndrome
D. All of the above

14. Anemia may be caused by:
A. Excessive bleeding
B. Decreased red blood cell production
C. Increased red blood cell destruction (hemolysis)
D. All of the above

15. Which cellular organelle listed below contains specialized enzymes whose functions involve hydrogen peroxide?
A. Mitochondria
B. Microbody

C. Nucleus
D. Golgi complex

16. Which genera of fungi listed below is not responsible for causing dermatophytosis?
A. Trichophyton
B. Microsporum
C. Histoplasma
D. Epidermophyton

17. The Ghon complex, a lesion in the lung and regional lymph nodes, is found in:
A. Actinomycosis
B. Primary tuberculosis
C. Blastomycosis
D. Histoplasmosis

18. Kidney stones (renal calculi) are a common complication in a patient with which disorder listed below?
A. Diabetes mellitus
B. Hyperthyroidism
C. Hyperparathyroidism
D. Hypopituitarism

19. Natural immunity (innate immunity) is resistance:
A. Acquired through contact with an antigen
B. Not acquired through contact with an antigen
C. Both of the above
D. None of the above

20. An injection of a drug into a patient who is allergic to this drug may lead to death due to:
A. Low levels of histamine
B. Hyperglobulinemia
C. Severe anaphylaxis (anaphylactic shock)
D. Localized anaphylaxis

21. The lipidoses are lipid storage disease caused by abnormalities in the enzymes that metabolize fat. They result in a toxic accumulation of fat by-products in tissue. Gaucher's diseases is a disorder of lipid metabolism caused by a deficiency of
A. Hexosaminidase A

B. Sphingomyelinase
C. Glucocerebrosidase
D. Alpha – L - iduronidase

22. All of the following statements concerning syphilis are true except :
A. It is a sexually transmitted disease caused by infection with treponema palidum (a spirochete)
B. Congenital infection in neonates and infants can occur.
C. It occurs in three stages: primary, secondary and tertiary
D. Gummas are lesions of primary syphilis
E. The prognosis is good if treated early, tertiary syphilis causes irreversible heart failure, dementia and disability
F. Parenteral penicillium G is the drug of choice for treating all stages.

23. Nephritic syndrome is a syndrome comprising the clinical symptoms of:
A. Nephritis
B. Hematuria
C. Hypertension
D. Renal failure
E. All of the above

24. Which of the following is a fungal infection that may develop in people who have poorly controlled diabetes?
A. Aspergillosis
B. Coccidioidomycosis
C. Mucormycosis
D. Crypttococcosis

25. Which type of leukemia listed below is the most common pediatric cancer?
A. Acute myeloid leukemia
B. Chronic myelocytic leukemia
C. Acute lymphocytic leukemia
D. Chronic lymphocytic leukemia

26. Which of the following are causes of ascites, the accumulation of fluid in the abdominal cavity?
A. Cirrhosis

B. Heart failure
C. Intra-abdominal cancer
D. Kidney failure
E. Tuberculosis
F. All of the above

27. Herpes Zoster (Shingles) is thought to be the adult counter - part of which of the following disease?
A. Rubella
B. Mumps
C. Smallpox
D. Chickenpox

28. Which type of Hepatitis is described below?
- It is spread by fecal-oral transmission; parenteral infection does not occur
- It has an incubation period of 21-45 days.
- It does not cause a chronic carrier state
- It is also called infectious hepatitis

A. Hepatitis A
B. Hepatitis B
C. Non A non B hepatitis
D. Hepatitis E

29. Which of the following is also known as Vincent infection or trench mouth?
A. Juvenile gingivitis
B. Desquamate gingivitis
C. Acute necrotizing ulcerative gingivitis (ANUG)
D. Rapidly progressing periodontitis

30. A 19 year old man suffering from non-suppurative enlargement of the parotid glands and painful swelling of the testes. He also complains of pain while eating, headache and general malaise. This man is most likely suffering from?
A. German measles (Rubella)
B. Measles (Rubeola)
C. Mumps
D. Common cold

E. Influenza
F. Pharyngitis

31. Kaposi's sarcoma, a malignant tumor of vascular organ that appear painless and purple raised patches on the skin, frequently is associated with

A. Diabetes
B. Chronic renal failure
C. AIDS
D. Hypertension

32. The primary inflection with herpes simplex virus is characterized by all of the following except :

A. Average course of 2-3 weeks
B. A few lesions on the lips or the mouth that resolve over a week to 10 days
C. Fever chills and malaise (flu-like-symptoms)
D. Vesicle formation

33. Which of the following skin growths closely resembles squamous cell carcinoma

A. Dermatofibromas
B. Seborrhea Keratosis
C. Achrochordon
D. Keratoacanthoma
E. Actinic keratosis

34. Which two antifungal agents listed are also referred to as polyene antibiotics ?

A. Nystatin
B. Miconazole
C. Flucytosine
D. Amphotericin
E. Ketoconazole

35. All of the following statements concerning malignant melanoma are true except :

A. It originates in the pigment-producing cells of the skin (melanocytes)
B. It is considered of be the most severe type of skin cancer
C. It is most common in fair skinned persons

D. It is most often associated with excessive exposure to sunlight
E. It rarely spreads (metastasizes to distant parts of the body)

36. All of the following bacteria have been found to be the principal bacteria associated with juvenile periodontitis except:
A. Actino-bacillius actino-mycetamcomitans (AA)
B. Capnocytophaga ochraceus
C. Wolinella recta
D. Prevotella intermedius
E. Eikenella corodens

37. Which of the following is the drug of choice for treating Candidiasis?
A. Penicillin
B. Cephalosporins
C. Clindamycin
D. Nystatin

38. Which syndrome listed below is condition affecting girls, in which, one of the two X chromosomes is partially or completely missing?
A. Klinefelter's syndrome
B. Triple X syndrome
C. Turner syndrome
D. Down's syndrome

39. Which of the flowing immunodeficiency disorders is the most serious ?
A. Wiskott - Aldrich syndrome
B. Severe combined immunodeficiency disease (SCID)
C. Ataxia - Telangiectasia
D. Hyper – IgE syndrome

40. Which of the following is the proper time and temperature for autoclaving?
A. 35° F for 1 hour
B. 25° F for 15-20 minutes
C. 450° F for 5 minutes
D. 89° F for 30 minutes

41. The area of the cytoplasm in prokaryotic cells in which DNA is located is called?

A. Granules
B. Nucleoid
C. Plastids
D. Transposons

42. All of the following statements concerning ethylene oxide sterilization are true except:

A. It is used extensively in hospitals for the sterilization of heat-sensitive materials such as surgical instrument and plastics
B. It kills by alkylating both proteins and nucleic acids
C. It is a fast process, 20 – 50 minutes depending on the material to sterilized
D. It is fairly toxic to humans and is also flammable

43 Gamma hemolytic streptococci can be differentiated from alpha & beta streptococci on blood agar plates by observing

A. A clear zone of hemloysis about the colony with no intact corpuscles
B. Small colonies surrounded by a greenish discoloration
C. No hemolysis
D. Small colonies surrounded by a zone of partial hemolyses and an outer clear zone

44. Which one of the following tests is abnormally prolonged in idiopathic thrombocytopenic purpura?

A. Partial thromb plastin time (PTT)
B. Thrombin time
C. Bleeding time
D. Prothrombin time (PT)

45. Acromegaly is

A. Excessive growth caused by the over-secretion of thyroid hormone
B. Excessive growth caused by the over-secretion of growth hormone
C. Excessive growth caused by the over-secretion of parathyroid hormone
D. Excessive growth caused by the over-secretion of epinephrine

46. Osgood - Schlatter disease is

A. Destruction of the growth plate in the neck of the thigh bone
B. Inflammation of the bone and cartilage at the top of the shinbone
C. A relatively common condition in which backache and humpback are caused by changes in the vertebrae
D. A rare form of inflammation of bone and cartilage affecting one of the small bones, the navicular bone, in the foot.

47. Which immunoglobulin antibody listed is some times referred to as the Secretory immunoglobulin?

A. Ig D
B. Ig E
C. Ig A
D. Ig M

48. All of the following abnormalities in parathyroid function are matched with the appropriate association except

A. Primary hyperparathyroidism; adenoma
B. Secondary hyperparathyroidism; liver disease
C. Tertiary hyperparathyroidism: hyperparathyroidism which persists after definitive therapy for secondary hyperparathyroidism.
D. Hypoparathyroidism; most commonly caused by accidental surgery excision during thyroidectomy
E. Pseudoparathyrodism: defective end organ responsiveness to PTH

49. Which of the following is the most important contributor to arterial thrombosis?

A. Pregnancy
B. Oral contraceptives
C. Atherosclerosis
D. Smoking

50. Generalized edema is known as:

A. Hydrothorax
B. Anasarca
C. Hydropericardium
D. Ascites

E. Exudate
F. Transudate

51. All of the following are amyloid-associated conditions, except:
A. Alzheimer's disease
B. Familial Mediterranean fever
C. Diabetes mellitus Type 2
D. Parkinson's disease
E. Senile amyloidosis

52. An infiltrate of which one of the following cells is most characteristic of the early stages of the acute inflammation?
A. Basophils
B. Eosinophils
C. Neutrophils
D. Monocytes

53. Which of the following is the most common type of peptic ulcer?
A. Esophageal ulcers
B. Gastric ulcers
C. Duodenal ulcers
D. Stress ulcers

54. Which type of necrosis listed below is the basic and most common type?
A. Liquefaction necrosis
B. Gangrenous necrosis
C. Caseous necrosis
D. Coagulative necrosis
E. Fat necrosis
F. Fibrinoid necrosis

55. The cause of most types of leukemia is:
A. Viral
B. Fungal
C. Bacterial
D. Unknown

56. The usual site of latency for the Herpes simplex virus type 2 is:

A. The cranial sensory ganglia
B. The lumbar or sacral sensory ganglia
C. The cranial or thoracic sensory ganglia
D. B - lymphocytes

57. Emphysema is associated with:

A. Pollutants
B. Genetic factors
C. Cigarette smoking
D. Infection
E. All of the above

58. Young plaque is dominated by which of bacteria listed below?

A. Gram-positive COCCI
B. Gram-positive rods
C. Gram-negative rods
D. Filaments

59. Which type of bronchogenic carcinoma listed below is the most aggressive?

A. Squamous cell carcinoma
B. Adenocarcinoma
C. Small cell (oat cell) carcinoma
D. Large cell carcinoma

60. Which of the following cancers is second in incidence only to carcinoma of the lung in men and third after breast and lung cancer in women?

A. Esophageal cancer
B. Stomach cancer
C. Colorectal cancer
D. Liver cancer

61. Which type of cancer listed below is the most common malignancy of women?

A. Bone cancer
B. Stomach cancer
C. Breast cancer
D. Ovarian cancer

62. Which of the following has been shown to be the most effective antimicrobial agent for reducing plaque and gingivitis long-term?

A. Stannous fluoride
B. Phenolic compounds
C. Chlorhexidine
D. Ouarternary ammonium compounds

63. Cephalosporins and penicillins both have which mode of action listed below?

A. Affect cell membrane
B. Interfere with protein synthesis
C. Affect cell wall
D. Interfere with normal biosynthetic pathways

64. Neoplastic epidermal cells, often with keratin pearls, characterize which type of skin cancer listed below?

A. Squamous cell carcinoma
B. Basal cell carcinoma
C. Malignant melanoma
D. None of the above

65. Which cells listed below are the most important phagocytic cells?

A. Eosinophils and basophils
B. Neutrophils and basophils
C. Neutrophils and macrophages
D. Macrophages and eosinophils

66. People with cystic fibrosis, burn victims, individuals with cancer, and patients requiring extensive stays in intensive care units are particularly at risk for infection with which species listed below?

A. Bacteroides
B. Fusobacterium
C. Pseudomonas
D. Streptococcus

67. A xenograft is:
A. A transfer of an individual's own tissue
B. A transfer of tissue between genetically identical individuals (identical twins)
C. A transfer of tissue between different species
D. A transfer of tissue between genetically different members of the same species (one human to another)

68. During phagocytosis, bacteria are ingested by the invagination of the neutrophil (PMN's) cell membrane around the bacteria to form a vacuole (phagosome). This engulfment is enhanced by the binding of IgG antibodies to the surface of the bacteria, a process called:
A. Transformation
B. Opsonization
C. Transduction
D. Recombination

69. An increase in the size of an organ or tissue due to an increase in the size of cells is known as
A. Hypertrophy
B. Atrophy
C. Hyperplasia
D. Hypoplasia
E. Metaplasia

70. Cytokines are soluble proteins secreted by which of the following cells?
A. Lymphocytes
B. Macrophages
C. Fibroblasts
D. Platelets
E. All of the above

71. Which myeloproliferative disorder listed below is characterized by an increased number of platelets?
A. Polycythemia vera
B. Myelofibrosis
C. Thrombocythemia
D. Chronic myelocytic leukemia

72. Histamine release within the body causes:

A. Increased capillary permeability
B. Increased gastric secretion
C. Bronchiolar constriction
D. Fall in blood pressure
E. All of the above

73. Carbon Monoxide

A. Attaches to the nucleus of red blood cells and blocks their capacity to replicate
B. Attaches to the cytoplasm membrane of red blood cells and causes lysis of the cell
C. Attaches to the hemoglobin of red blood cells and blocks their capacity to carry oxygen
D. Attaches t the cell membrane of red blood cells blocks their capacity to move within vessels

74. The most common bone lesion is a (an)

A. Osteochondroma
B. Fractures
C. Osteoma
D. Osteoblastoma

75. When gallstones are in the gallbladder the condition is know as:

A. Choledocholithiasis
B. Cholesterolosis, strawberry gall bladder
C. Cholelithiasis
D. Divertiuculosis of the gallbladder

76. All of the following statements concerning B cells are true except :

A. They mature in the bone marrow and migrate to lymphoid organs
B. They are found in the germinal centers of the spleen and lymph nodes
C. They are progenitors of plasma cells.
D. They involve in humoral antibody mediated and cell mediated immunity

E. They function to search out identity and bind with specific antigens

77. A serious condition in which the quantity of blood pumped by heart each minute (cardiac output) is insufficient to meet body normal requirements for oxygen and nutrients is called

A. Heart bock
B. Ventricular tachycardia
C. Congestive heart failure
D. Atrial fibrillation

78. Which of the following is the most frequently employed diagnostic laboratory technique for the microscopic detection of antigens in tissue secretion or in cell suspensions?

A. Immuofluorescence (Fluorescent antibody)
B. Agglutination
C. Radiommunoassay
D. Precipitation (Precepitin)
E. Enzyme Liked Immunosorbent Assay (ELISA)

79. Diabetes mellitus type –2 associated with all of the following characteristics except

A. Normal or increased insulin syntheses
B. Onset in adulthood
C. Autoimmune origin
D. Associated with obesity
E. Rare ketoacidosis

80. All of the following are characteristic of an exudates except:

A. Protein-rich
B. Low specific gravity
C. Glucose-poor
D. Cell-rich

81. Brief loss of consciousness and sometimes memory after an injury to the brain that doesn't cause obvious physical damage is called a

A. Hematoma
B. Infarction
C. Concussion
D. Meningioma

82. Malignant nephrosclerosis is a condition associated with
A. Server Hyperlipidemia
B. Severe high blood pressure
C. Severe hyper-albuminemia
D. Severe low blood pressure

83. Which of the following is the most common inherited disease leading to death among white people in the United States?
A. von Hippel Lindau disease
B. Cystic fibrosis
C. Marfan's syndrome
D. Familial hypercholesterolemia

84. All of the following statements concerning the rubella virus are true except:
A. It is a member of the toga virus family and is an enveloped virus; comprise of an icosahedral nucleocapsid and a positive–stranded single stranded RNA genome
B. It causes rubella (German Measles) and congenital rubella syndrome
C. It is transmitted by the bite of a rabid animal
D. Prevention involves immunization with the live, attenuated vaccine

85. Chronic bronchitis is primarily a disease of:
A. Alcoholics
B. Cigarette smokers
C. Miners
D. Patients with a family history of allergy

86. The cytopathic effect that is seen when a virus infects a specific cell culture
A. Is the same for most viruses
B. Is not useful in diagnostic virology
C. Is characteristic of each virus and can be used for detection of that virus
D. Does not affect the specific infected cells.

87. Acquired immunodeficiency syndrome (AIDS) is caused by an enveloped single stranded, linear, positive polarity RNA virus known as :

A. An arbovirus
B. A parvovirus
C. A retrovirus
D. An adenovirus

88. All of the following viruses are paramyxoviruses except:
A. Mumps virus
B. Measles virus
C. Influenza A, B, and C viruses
D. Respiratory syncytial virus (RSV)
E. Parainfluenza virus

89. Infections caused by certain nematodes cause
A. Marked neutrophilia
B. Marked eosinophilia
C. Marked basophilia
D. All of the above

90. Which of the following types of lymphoma is distinguished by a particular kind of cancer cell called a Reed – Sternberg cell which has a distinctive appearance under microscope?
A. Non –Hodgkin's lymphoma
B. Burkitt's lymphoma
C. Hodgkin's disease
D. Mycosis Fungicides

91. Which of the following is a powerful oxidizing agent that inactivates bacteria and most viruses by oxidizing free sulfhydryl groups?
A. Alcohol
B. Chlorine
C. Formaldehyde
D. Phenol

92. Two different pathways are involved in the metabolism of glucose one - anaerobic and one aerobic; the anaerobic process occurs in the
A. Mitochondria and is very efficient
B. Cytoplasm and is only moderately efficient
C. Mitochondria and is not efficient
D. Cytoplasm and is very efficient

93. A cell wall that contains teichoic acids and a thick peptido-glycans (murein) layer is characteristic of

A. Viruses
B. Gram positive bacteria
C. Fungi
D. Gram negative bacteria

94. Vaccines that contain a live virus whose pathogenicity has been attenuated are used against all of the following diseases except:

A. Measles
B. Mumps
C. Rabies
D. Rubella

95. Viruses that infect bacteria are known as :

A. Protoplasts
B. Saprophytes
C. Bacteriophages
D. Commensals

96. A laceration of the esophagus and the upper part of the stomach during forceful vomiting, retching, or hiccups is called:

A. Hiatal-Hernia
B. Mallory-Weiss syndrome
C. Achalasia
D. Acid reflux syndrome

97. All these organs get usually damaged from prolonged hypertension except?

A. Kidneys
B. Heart
C. Stomach
D. Brain

98. Which glands listed below fail to develop in children with the DiGeorge's anomaly (DiGeorge's syndrome)?

A. Thyroid gland
B. Thymus gland

C. Pituitary gland
D. Parathyroid glands
E. Adrenal glands

99. All of the following conditions are associated with a prolonged bleeding time except:
A. Idiopathic thrombocytopenic purpura
B. Von Willebrand's disease
C. Hemophilia
D. Patents taking anticoagulants (e.g. dicumarol, heparin etc.)
E. Long term treatment with aspirin

100. All of the following are examples of Type III hypersensitivity reactions (immune complex) except:
A. Arthus reaction
B. Farmer's lung
C. Myasthenia gravis
D. Cheesemaker's lung
E. Serum sickness
F. Rheumatoid arthritis

Answer Key to MCQs in Microbiology and Pathology Part I

1	C	2	B	3	C	4	D
5	C	6	C	7	C	8	E
9	C	10	B	11	B	12	D
13	A	14	D	15	B	16	C
17	B	18	C	19	B	20	C
21	C	22	D	23	E	24	C
25	C	26	F	27	D	28	A
29	C	30	C	31	C	32	D
33	D	34	A, D	35	E	36	C
37	D	38	C	39	B	40	B
41	B	42	C	43	C	44	C
45	B	46	B	47	C	48	B
49	C	50	B	51	D	52	C
53	C	54	D	55	D	56	B
57	E	58	A	59	C	60	C
61	C	62	C	63	C	64	A
65	C	66	C	67	C	68	B
69	A	70	E	71	C	72	E
73	C	74	B	75	C	76	D
77	C	78	A	79	C	80	B
81	C	82	B	83	B	84	C
85	B	86	C	87	C	88	C
89	B	90	C	91	B	92	B
93	B	94	C	95	C	96	B
97	C	98	B, D	99	C	100	C

Part II

1. Which of the following is the most common cause of sudden, severe abdominal pain and abdominal surgery?

A. Ulcerative colitis
B. Acute appendicitis
C. Crohn's disease
D. Carcinoid tumor

2. Swollen bleeding gums accompanied by muscle joint and bone pain are characteristic of:

A. Pellagra
B. Scurvy
C. Beri-beri
D. Rickets

3. The main advantage of active immunity is that resistance is:

A. Available immediately
B. Short Term
C. Long term
D. None of the above

4. Which two enzymes listed below would be evaluated in the blood of a patient suffering from acute pancreatitis?

A. Alkaline phosphates
B. Acid phosphates
C. Lipase
D. Amylase
E. SGOT / SGPT

5. Three species of bacteria account for more than 80% of all cases of bacterial meningitis. Which species listed below is not one of them?

A. Neisseria meningitis
B. Hemophilus influenzae
C. Staphylococcus aureus
D. Sterptococcus pneumoniae

6. **Urolithiasis is a condition resulting from the presence or formation of calculi in the urinary tract. Most of these calculi are:**
   A. Ammonium magnesium phosphate stones
   B. Calcium stones
   C. Uric acid stones
   D. Cystine stones

7. **Aflatoxins are produced by**
   A. Candida species
   B. Coccidioides species
   C. Aspergillus species
   D. Histoplasma species

8. **Jaundice refers to yellow discoloration of the skin, sclera and tissues caused by**
   A. Hyperlipidemia
   B. Hyperglycemia
   C. Hyperbilirubinemia
   D. Hypocalcaemia

9. **The most common cause of cirrhosis is :**
   A. Wilson's disease
   B. Alcohol abuse
   C. Bile duct obstruction
   D. Hemochromatosis

10. **Which species listed below has been implicated in the dental caries process?**
    A. Staphylococcus
    B. Bacteroides
    C. E. coli
    D. Streptococcus

11. **Which growth curve listed below describes the lytic reproduction cycle that releases a large number of phage simultaneously**
    A. One step growth curve
    B. Two step growth curve
    C. Horizontal growth curve
    D. None of the above

12. Which system below is concerned chiefly with phagocytes and antibody formations?

A. Muscular system
B. Nervous system
C. Reticulo-endothelial system
D. Reticular activating system

13. All of the following statements concerning herpes simplex type 1 are true except:

A. Many children have a symptomatic primary infections
B. May be diagnosed by a Tzanck smear for rapid identification when skin lesions are involved
C. May involve a primary infection (e.g gingivo-stomatitis) or a recurrent infection (e.g. cold cores)
D. Can be treated prophylactically by vaccine

14. Which of the following is a neoplasm derived from all three germ cell layers?

A. Carcinoma
B. Sarcoma
C. Teratoma
D. APU Doma

15. The desired results in all surgical incisions is healing by :

A. Primary intention
B. Secondary intention
C. Tertiary intention
D. None of the above

16. Which cells listed below help to assist other T - cells and B - cells to express their immune function?

A. Cytotoxic (killer) cells
B. Plasma cells
C. T - helper cells
D. T - suppressor cells

17. All of the following are benign neoplasms except:

A. Papilloma
B. Adenoma
C. Sarcoma
D. Lipoma

18. Lactobacillus species are:
A. Gram negative rods that tend to form clusters
B. Gram negative cocci that tend to form clusters
C. Gram positive cocci that tend to form chains
D. Gram positive rods that tend to form chains

19. Which antibiotic listed below would be indicated for a patient requiring the administration of prophylactic antibiotic prior to dental treatment?
A. Tetracycline
B. Lincomycin
C. Amoxicilin
D. Chloramphenicol

20. All of the following are possible causes of tetany except:
A. Hypoparathyroidism
B. Rickets (Vitamin D deficiency)
C. Hypertension
D. Hyperventilation
E. Uremia

21. All of the following statements concerning X-linked agammaglobulinemia/Bruton's agammalobulinemia are true except:
A. It affects only boys
B. Result in decreased numbers or absence of B lymphocytes
C. Result in very low levels of antibodies
D. There is impaired resistance to viral infections
E. There is normal circulating T cells lymphocytes

22. The only *cold sterilizer solution* capable of destroying bacterial spores, viruses and vegetative bacteria is:
A. Quaternary ammonium compounds
B. Chlorhexidine
C. 90% isopropyl alcohol
D. 2% glutaraldehyde

23. All of the following bacteria produce a toxin that can be detected using the ELISA assay except.
A. E. coli
B. Vibrio cholera

C. Bacteroides
D. Staphylococcus aureus

24. Which type of pathogens provide the ultimate test for efficacy of sterilization?
A. Bacteria
B. Spore-forming
C. Virus
D. Fungi

25. All of the following species are found in saliva except
A. Actinomyces
B. Veillonella
C. Streptococcus
D. Staphylococcus

26. Anemia in a newborn can result form
A. Excessive blood loss during delivery
B. Excessive destruction of red blood cells
C. Impaired production of red blood cells
D. All of the above

27. Of the three types thyroiditis listed below, which one is the most common and the most common cause of hypothyroidism?
A. Hashimoto's thyroiditis
B. Sub acute granulomatous thyroiditis
C. Silent lympocyytic thyroiditis
D. All of the above

28. Which of the following is also known as marble bone disease or disease Albers - schonburg disease?
A. Fibrous dysplasia
B. Osteogenesis imperfecta
C. Osteopetrosis
D. Achondroplasia

29. Leukotriene C 4, D 4 and E 4 are collectively known as
A. Histamine
B. Slow reacting substances of anaphylaxis (SRS-A)

C. Heparin
D. Serotonin

30. Which of the following is an acute, self limited disease that occurs 6 - 8 days after the injection of a foreign protein (bovine albumin) and is characterized by fever, arthralgias, vasculitis and an acute glomerulonephritis?
A. Arthus reaction
B. Polyarteritis nodosa
C. Serum sickness
D. Systemic lupus Erythematosus

31. Which type of stock listed below most often associated with severe trauma to the CNS?
A. Hypovolemic shock
B. Cardiogenic shock
C. Septic Shock
D. Neurogenic Shock
E. Anaphylactic Shock

32. Which type of hypersensitive reaction listed below is characterized by a specific cytotropic antibody (IgE) that binds to receptors on basophils and mast cells and reacts with a specific antigen
A. Type I
B. Type II
C. Type III
D. Type IV

33. A nuclear change that involves the condensation and shrinkage of the cell nucleus with chromatin clumping is known as:
A. Pyknosis
B. Karyopyknosis
C. Karyolysis
D. Karyorrhexis

34. Impetigo (pyoderma) is a localized intraepidermal infection of the skin that is caused by
A. Streptococcus mutans and staphylococci epidermis
B. Streptococcus mitis & staphylococcus saprophyticus

C. Streptococcus pyogenes and staphylococcus aureus
D. Streptococcus pneumoniae and staphyloccous aureus

35. Gas gangrene is also called what?
A. Anthrax
B. Diphtheria
C. Myonecrosis
D. Pseudomebranous colitis

36. Which of the following statements is true concerning chronic leukemias?
A. They progress rapidly
B. They have a shorter, more devastating clinical course than the acute leukemias
C. They are characterized by proliferations of lymphoid or hematopoietic cells that are more mature than those of the acute leukemias
D. They constitute 75 % of all leukemias

37. Which group of viruses listed below possesses an RNA genome that does not function as positive or negative sense molecule but acts as a template for the viral DNA?
A. Corona viruses
B. Picorna viruses
C. Retro viruses
D. Toga viruses

38. The average age of people who have chronic lymphocytic leukemia (CLL) is
A. 10 years old
B. 25 years old
C. 45 Years old
D. 60 Years Old

39. All of the following diseases are associated with adenoviruses except:
A. Acute respiratory infections
B. Acute contagious conjunctivitis (pink eye)
C. Generalized systemic disease with a maculo-papular rash
D. Pharyngo-conjunctival fever characterized by fever, pharyngitis, and conjunctivitis

40. All of the following are benign tumors of mesenchymal origin except

A. Leomyoma
B. Rhabdomyoma
C. Osteosarcoma
D. Fibroma
E. Chondroma

41. All of the following bacteria may be etiologically related to dental caries except:

A. Streptococcus mutans
B. Actinomyces viscous
C. Acitnobacillus actinomycetamcomitans
D. Streptococcus salivarius
E. Streptococcus sanguis

42. A single - celled parasite that causes amoebiasis in humans is:

A. Giardia lamblia
B. Entamoeba histolytica
C. Trachomonas vaginalis
D. Balantidium coli

43. The large majority (90%) of cancers of the lung are a consequence of:

A. Hereditary factors
B. Alcohol consumption
C. Cigarette smoking
D. Diet

44. Alcohol requires which concentration listed below to kill bacteria, given sufficient time?

A. 10% - 20%
B. 30% - 40%
C. 50% - 60%
D. 70% - 95%

45. Which of these bacteria are the principle bacteria associated with acute necrotizing ulcerative gingivitis / ANUG?

A. Streptococcus sanguis
B. Prevotella intermedia

C. Spirochetes
D. Actinomyces israeli
E. Porphyromonas gingivalis

46. Mycobacterium cell walls contain a waxy substance composed of:
A. Resin acids
B. Chenic acids
C. Mycolic acids
D. Chenodeoxycholic acids

47. Which of the following are used in protective vaccines because of their antigenicity but have lost their toxicity?
A. Antitoxins
B. Toxoids
C. Mycotoxins
D. Endotoxins

48. All of the following bacteria have been found to be the principal bacteria associated with adult periodontitis except:
A. Porphyromonas gingivalis
B. Prevotella intermedia
C. Capnocytophaga ochraceus
D. Bacteroides forsythus
E. Campylobactor rectus

49. The rabies vaccine and clostridium tetani vaccine result in:
A. Naturally acquired passive immunity
B. Naturally acquired active immunity
C. Artificially acquired active immunity
D. Artificially acquired passive immunity

50. Renin is produced in the:
A. Liver
B. Intestines
C. Kidneys
D. Lungs

51. Pernicious anaemia is a megaloblastic anemia caused by the lack of
A. Vitamin C

B. Vitamin A
C. Vitamin B12
D. Vitamin K

52. All of the following statements concerning Peutz – Jeghers syndrome are true except :
A. It is a hereditary condition in which many small lumps called Juvenile polyps appear in a variety of sites in the GI tract, most commonly in the small intestine, esp in the jejunum
B. It only·affect males
C. It is characterized by melanin pigmentation of the oral mucosa especially of the lips and gingiva
D. People with this syndrome are at increased risk for cancer of the pancreas, breast, lung, ovary and uterus.

53. The most common cause of secondary hypertension is
A. Hormonal disorder
B. Kidney disease
C. Drugs
D. Congenital anomalies

54. All of the following cells have the ability to retain a latent capacity for mitotic division except:
A. Bone marrow cells
B. Liver cells
C. Blood cells
D. Neurons in the brain or spiral cord

55. All of the following are clinical features of hyperthyroidism except:
A. Restlessness, irritability and fatigability
B. Heat intolerance (sweating) due to increased SMR
C. Tachycardia (a rapid heart rate)
D. Weight gain
E. Fine hair
F. Diarrhoea
G. Tremor (shakiness)

56. All of the following features are of rheumatoid arthritis except:
A. Serum anti – IgG antibodies ie rhematoid factors

B. Osteophyte formation
C. Subcutaneous rheumatoid nodules
D. Fatigue, malaise, anorexia, weight gain, fever and myalgias.
E. Symmetric polyarthritis

57. Reye's syndrome is a serious and potentially fatal complication that occurs most commonly in children during epidemics of
A. Mumps
B. Measles
C. Influenza – B
D. Common cold

58. All of the following are the motor symptoms / changes in the motor functions in multiple sclerosis condition except:
A. Tremors
B. Weakness, clumsiness
C. Difficulty in walking or maintaining balance
D. Double vision
E. Diarrhoea
F. Stiffness, unsteadiness and unusual tiredness

59. A small foreign molecule that is not immunogenic by itself but can react with specific antibody is called a / an :
A. Epitope
B. Hapten
C. Plasmid
D. Immunogen

60. The biologic consequences of compliment activation include
A. Chemotaxis of phagocytes
B. Immune adherence and opsonization
C. Anaphylatoxin activity
D. Membrane activity
E. All of the above

61. Pyelonephritis most commonly occurs as result of a (an)
A. Oral cavity infection
B. Urinary tract infection
C. Skin infection
D. Pulmonary infection

62. All of the following statements concerning fungal spores are true except:

A. Morphologic characteristics (e.g. the shape, color and arrangement) of conidia are useful and for the identification of fungi.
B. A fungal spore is as resistant to heat as bacterial spores
C. Fungal spores cause allergies in some people
D. A conidium is an asexually formed fungal spore.

63. Which of the following make up the triad of findings found in Sjogren's syndrome?

A. Associated connective tissue disorders e.g. rheumatoid arthritis
B. Xerostomia, dry mouth
C. Diabetes
D. Nephrosclerosis
E. Cirrhosis of the liver
F. Keratoconjunctivitis Sicca ie dry eyes

64. All of the following bacteria are negative, facultatively anaerobic rods except

A. Escherichia
B. Salmonella
C. Streptococcus
D. Proteus

65. Another name for acute glomerulo-nephritis is

A. Rapidly progressive glomerulonephritis
B. Goodpasture's syndrome
C. Post- streptococcal glomerulonephritis
D. Alport's syndrome

66. Which type of Hepatitis is described below?

- The three main modes of transmission are via blood, during sexual intercourse and parentally from mother to newborn
- It has an incubation period averaging 60-90 days
- It can result in a carrier state or chronic liver disease
- It also called Serum Hepatitis

A. Hepatitis A
B. Hepatitis B

C. Hepatitis C
D. Hepatitis D

67. A bacteriophage with the ability to form a stable, non – disruptive relationship within bacterium is called a :

A. Virulent phage
B. Plasmid
C. Temperate phage
D. Phage T4

68. Which virus listed below shows changes in the antigenicity of its hemagglutinin and neuramindase proteins?

A. Mumps virus
B. Measles Virus
C. Influenza Virus
D. Epstein Barr virus

69. All of the following statements concerning basal cell carcinoma are true, except

A. It is by far the most common malignant tumor of the skin
B. It originates in the lowest layer of the epidermis (Basel cell layer)
C. Usually develops on skin surface that are exposed to sunlight
D. Rather than spreading to distant parts of the body, it usually invades and destroys the surrounding tissues.
E. It is rarely cured by surgical resection

70. The infectious viral particle is called a

A. Viroid .
B. Virion
C. Prion
D. Neon

71. Differentiation is a measure of a tumor's resemblance to normal tissue. Anaplasia is

A. A high degree of differentiation
B. A moderate degree of differentiation
C. The absence of differentiation
D. Total differentiation

72. All of the following tissues regenerate except:
A. Bone
B. Intestinal mucosa
C. Liver
D. Striated muscle
E. Cartilage

73. The food and drug administration recommends the use of which antibiotic listed below to be reserved for serious anaerobic infections ?
A. Penicillin V
B. Tetracycline
C. Clindamycin
D. Cephalosporins

74. Most prominent symptoms of a pheochromocytoma is:
A. Diarrhea
B. Internal bleeding
C. High blood pressure
D. Hypoglycemia

75. The primary acidogenic microorganisms in the oral cavity are
A. Spirochetes
B. Streptococcus
C. Fusobacterium
D. Lactobacillus

76. Pseudomembranous colitis is a sign of toxicity for which antibiotic listed below ?
A. Cephalosporins
B. Tetracycline
C. Clindamycin
D. Carbenicillin

77. Which of the following is the proper time and temperature for dry heat sterilization?
A. 3200 F/160 C for 2 hours
B. 2500 for 20-30 minutes
C. 4500 F for 5 minutes
D. 890 F for 30 minutes

78. The enterotoxin produced by staphylococcus aureus causes
A. Bacterial dysentery
B. Gas gangrene
C. Food poisoning
D. Scarlet fever

79. The killing or removal of all microorganisms including bacterial spores is called?
A. Disinfection
B. Cleaning
C. Sterilization
D. Wiping

80. During which growth phase of the typical growth curve of a bacterial culture is the cell increasing in mass or cell number?
A. Lag phase
B. Log phase
C. Secondary phase
D. Death phase

81. Osteomyelitis is a bone infection usually caused by:
A. Parasites
B. Viruses
C. Bacteria
D. Fungi

82. All of the following statements concerning erythema multiforme are true except
A. It is a disorder characterized by patches of red raised skin that often look like targets and are usually distributed symmetrically over the body
B. It is usually a reaction to a drug, most often penicillins or infectious agent and is commonly associated with herpes simplex infection
C. It is an uncommon disorder with a peak incidence in the first decade of life
D. It usually heals on its own but Stevens Johnson syndrome (Which is a very severe form) can be fatal

83. Paget's disease of bone / osteitis deformans is characterized by :

A. High serum calcium, low serum phosphate, high serum alkaline phosphatase
B. Normal serum calcium, phosphorous and alkaline phosphatase
C. Normal serum calcium and phosphorus with a markedly increased serum alkaline phosphatase
D. Normal serum phosphorus, low serum calcium, high serum alkaline phosphatase

84. Which blood group listed below has neither antigen A or B?

A. A
B. B
C. O
D. AB

85. Characteristics of systemic lupus erythematosus include all of the following except:

A. "Butterfly rash" on the face
B. Skin rash
C. Sensitivity to light
D. Fluid around the lungs, heart or other organs
E. Blindness
F. Arthritis
G. Kidney, nerve, or brain dysfunction

86. Metabolic acidosis occurs in which stage of shock?

A. Non-progressive (early) stage
B. Progressive stage
C. Irreversible stage
D. May occur in any stage

87. An embolus is usually:

A. Fat
B. Amniotic fluid
C. A blood clot
D. An air bubble

88. Which of the following is the classic lesion of rheumatic fever

A. The Barr body
B. The brush field body

C. The Aschoff body
D. The charcot - Leyden body

89. Anaphylatoxins
A. Produce inflammation
B. Cause enhanced capillary permeability
C. Induce smooth muscle contraction
D. Cause hypertension
E. All of the above

90. An abscess is
A. Tumor composed of granulation tissue
B. An abnormal sac containing air or fluid
C. An accumulation of pus
D. Considered to be pre-malignant

91. Decreased melanin pigmentation is seen in
A. Addison's disease
B. Jaundice
C. Albinism and vitiligo
D. Hemosiderosis

92. Granulomatous inflammation is typical of the tissue response elicited by all of the following except:
A. Fungal infections
B. Tuberculosis
C. Acute meningitis
D. The presence of foreign material e.g. suture or talc
E. Leprosy
F. Sarcoidosis

93. A specific chromosome marker characterizes which type of leukemia listed bellow:
A. Acute lymphocytic leukemia
B. Chronic myelocytic leukemia
C. Acute myeloid leukemia
D. Chronic lymphocytic leukemia

94. All of the following are RNA enveloped viruses except
A. Picorna-viruses
B. Human immunodeficiency virus (HIV)

C. Measles, mumps, rubella and hepatitis - C viruses
D. Respiratory viruses

95. Chronic obstructive pulmonary disease COPD is a group of disorders characterized by airflow obstruction during respiration. Which one those listed below is marked by dyspnea and wheezing expiration caused by episodic narrowing of the airways?
A. Bronchial asthma
B. Chronic bronchitis
C. Emphysema
D. Bronchiectasis

96. Which of the following DNA enveloped viruses are the largest and most complex?
A. Herpes viruses
B. Hepatitis B virus
C. Pox viruses
D. Rabies virus

97. A malignant tumor of skeletal muscle is know as ?
A. A fibroma
B. A rhabdomyosarcoma
C. A rhabdomyoma
D. A leiomyoma

98. The principal oral site for the growth of spirochetes, fusobacteria and other gram negative anaerobes is
A. Saliva
B. Calculus
C. The gingival margin
D. The gingival sulcus

99. Which of the following can cause mutation?
A. Ultraviolet light
B. Chemicals
C. Radiations
D. Viruses
E. All of the above

100. Which antibiotic listed below is considered to be a broad spectrum antibiotics?

A. Ampicillin
B. Penicillin G
C. Cephalosporins
D. Penicillin V

Answer Key to MCQs in Microbiology and Pathology Part II

1	B	2	B	3	C	4	C,D
5	C	6	B	7	C	8	C
9	B	10	D	11	A	12	C
13	D	14	C	15	A	16	C
17	C	18	D	19	C	20	C
21	D	22	D	23	C	24	B
25	D	26	D	27	A	28	C
29	B	30	C	31	D	32	A
33	A	34	C	35	C	36	C
37	C	38	D	39	C	40	C
41	C	42	B	43	C	44	D
45	B, C	46	C	47	B	48	C
49	C	50	C	51	C	52	B
53	B	54	D	55	D	56	B
57	C	58	E	59	B	60	E
61	B	62	B	63	A,B,F	64	C
65	C	66	B	67	C	68	C
69	E	70	B	71	C	72	D
73	C	74	C	75	B	76	C
77	A	78	C	79	C	80	B
81	C	82	C	83	C	84	C
85	E	86	B	87	C	88	C
89	E	90	C	91	C	92	C
93	B	94	A	95	A	96	C
97	B	98	D	99	E	100	C

Part III

1. **Which subtypes of non-Hodgkin's lymphoma listed below closely linked to the Epstein Barr virus ?**
   A. Mycosis fungicides
   B. Burkitt's lymphoma
   C. None of the above
   D. Both of the above

2. **Various strains of which species listed below produce the enzyme penicillinase:**
   A. Streptococcus
   B. Pseudomonas
   C. Staphylococcus
   D. Mycobacterium

3. **Which malabsorption syndrome listed below is an inherited disorder in which an allergic intolerance to gluten, a protein, cause changes in the intestine that result in malabsorption**
   A. Tropical sprue
   B. Celiac disease
   C. Intestine lymphangiectasia
   D. Whipple disease

4. **Transcription**
   A. Is the synthesis of mRNA from RNA by RNA dependent DNA polymerase
   B. Is the synthesis of mRNA from DNA by RNA dependent DNA polymerase
   C. IS the synthesis of mRNA from DNA by DNA dependent RNA polymerase
   D. IS the synthesis of mRNA from RNA by RNA dependent RNA polymerize

5. **Mis-sense mutations**
   A. Stop protein synthesis prematurely
   B. Result in the substitution of one amino acid for another
   C. Generates a termination codon
   D. Almost always destroy protein function

6. Endotoxins are the lipopolysaccharide component of the cell wall of

A. Gram-positive bacteria
B. Gram negative bacteria
C. Mycoplasma
D. Viruses

7. All of the following statements concerning serotonin are true except

A. It is widely considered to be a neurotransmitter
B. It is present in the brain
C. It is believed to play a role in temperature regulation sensory perception and in the onset of sleep
D. It is synthesized from the amino acid argenine

8. All of the following concerning sickle cell anemia are true except:

A. It is an inherited condition characterized by sickle shaped red blood cells and chronic hemolytic anemia
B. The red blood cells contain an abnormal form of hemoglobin that reduces the amount of oxygen in the cells causing them to become crescent or sickle shaped
C. It affects whites almost exclusively
D. The sickle shaped cells block and damage the capillaries in the spleen, kidneys, brain, bones and other organs reducing their oxygen supply

9. Osteomalacia is caused by a :

A. Vitamin B deficiency in adults
B. Vitamin C deficiency in children
C. Vitamin D deficiency in adults
D. Vitamin A deficiency in children

10. All of the following are characteristics of gout except

A. Most often affects the joint at the base of the big toe, condition called podagra
B. Higher incidence in women
C. Hard lumps of urate crystals (tophi) are deposited under the skin around joints

D. An abnormally high uric acid level in the blood (hyperuricemia)

11. Hay fever and allergies to certain foods are examples of :

A. Antibody dependent cytotoxic hypersensitivity reactions
B. Immune complex mediated hypersensitivity reactions
C. Atopic allergies
D. Cell mediated or delayed hypersensitivity reactions

12. All of the following statements concerning infectious mononucleosis are true except:

A. It is caused by the Epstein bar versus (EBV)
B. It is a disease of old age
C. It is sometime called kissing disease
D. It is associated with the production of typical lymphocytes and IgM heterophile antibodies identified by the heterophile test

13. Which of the following is the most common cause of death in the early hours following the onset of a myocardial infarction/ heart attack ?

A. Cardiogenic shock
B. Arrhythmias
C. Ventricular rupture
D. Mural thrombosis

14. The most serious complication of pericarditis is

A. Infection
B. Fever
C. Cardiac tamponade
D. Leukocytosis

15. Which of the following is the most common joint disorder?

A. Rheumatoid arthritis
B. Psoriatic arthritis
C. Osteoarthritis
D. Systemic lupus erythematosus
E. Discoid lupus erythematosus

16. An infection is epidemic if:

A. It has a worldwide distribution

B. It is constantly present at a low level in a specific population
C. It occurs much more frequently than usual
D. It is highly communicable

17. The characteristic cell components of chronic inflammation include all of the following except:
A. Lymphocytes
B. Plasma cells
C. Polymorphonuclear leukocytes
D. Macrophages

18. Which of the following may cause blood in the urine / hematuria?
A. Bladder or kidney disease
B. Glomerulonephritis
C. Kidney stones
D. Kidney cysts
E. Sickle cell anemia
F. Hydronephrosis
G. All of the above

19. Which cystic disease of the kidney listed below is the most common inherited disorder of the kidney?
A. Adult polycystic kidney disease
B. Infantile pilocystic kidney disease
C. Medullary cystic disease
D. Medullary sponge kidney

20. Which of the following is most commonly caused by left ventricular failure (congestive heart failure)?
A. Bronchiectasis
B. Chronic bronchitis
C. Ateclectasis
D. Pulmonary edema

21. Which of the following predispose people to pneumonia?
A. Alcoholism
B. Cigarette smoking
C. Diabetes
D. Heart failure

E. Chronic objectives pulmonary disease (COPD)
F. All of the above

22. Usually the main symptoms of lung cancers
A. A persistent cough
B. Diarrhea
C. A low grade fever
D. A skin rash

23. Lymphomas principally involve which of the following
A. Lymph nodes
B. Spleen
C. Liver
D. Bone narrow
E. All of the above

24. Which type of cancer listed below is the second most common cause of cancer death?
A. Liver cancer
B. Bone cancer
C. Prostate cancer
D. Testicular cancer

25. Which two antibiotics listed below are usually prescribed in the treatment of Rickettsial disease?
A. Tetracycline
B. Polymixin B
C. Erythromycin
D. Chloramphenicol

26. Which term listed below is an interactive associations between two populations of different species living together, in which one population benefits from the association while the other is not affected—
A. Latency
B. Mutualism
C. Symbiosis
D. Commensalisms

27. Which toxin or enzyme listed below produced by Group A Streptococcus (S pyogenes) activates plasminogen to form plasmin which dissolves fibrin in clots, thrombi and emboli?
A. Streptokinase
B. Streptodornase
C. Hyaluronidase
D. Erythrogenic toxin
E. Streptolysin O

28. Freund's adjuvant is a mixture composed of
A. Mineral oil
B. Lanolin
C. Killed mycobacteria
D. All of the above

29. All of the following are formed via the cyclo-oxygenase pathway except
A. Prostaglandins
B. Prostacyclin
C. Leukotrienes
D. Thromboxanes

30. All of the following are considered to be the risk factors for developing atherosclerosis except
A. Increased age
B. High blood cholesterol levels
C. Diabetes
D. Smoking
E. Drug use

31. Lysozyme degrades
A. Peptidoglycans
B. RNA – polymerase
C. Lipopolysaccharide
D. Chitin

32. Very severe hypothyroidism in adults is called?
A. Cretinism
B. Plummer's Syndrome
C. Myxoedema
D. Graves disease

33. Which cellular organelle listed below contains digestive enzymes?

A. Ribosome
B. Inclusions
C. Lysosome
D. Mitochondria

34. All of the following statements concerning Ludwig's angina are true, except:

A. Most cases appear to be a mixed infection
B. It is often caused by normal oral flora gaining access through an infected tooth
C. It can cause severe swelling in the floor of the mouth, even forcing the tongue upward blocking the airway
D. Fever and malaise are usually not present

35. The classic symptom of coronary artery disease is:

A. Coughing
B. Venous congestion
C. Angina pectoris
D. Dizziness

36. Rheumatic fever is:

A. Inflammation of joints (arthritis) and the spleen (splenomegaly) resulting from a staphylococcal infection, usually of the throat
B. Inflammation of joints (arthritis) and the parotid glands (parotitis) resulting from a streptococcal infection, usually of the middle ear
C. Inflammation of the joints (arthritis) and the heart (carditis) resulting from a streptococcal infection, usually of the throat
D. Inflammation of the joints (arthritis) and the thyroid gland (goiter) resulting from a staphylococcal infection, usually of the blood

37. Which type of infection listed below often causes leukocytosis?

A. Parasitic
B. Viral
C. Bacterial
D. Fungal

38. The vascular phase of the acute inflammation involves all of the following cells except:
A. Platelets
B. Tissue mast cells
C. Eosinophils
D. Basophils

39. The increased excretion of calcium in the kidneys results in:
A. Jaundice
B. Nephrolithiasis
C. Polycystic kidney disease
D. Diabetes

40. Who would be at risk for black lung disease?
A. Aerospace workers
B. Farmers
C. Coal workers
D. Sandstone or granite cutters

41. Infection with the Epstein-Barr virus can cause infectious mononucleosis, which may be characterized by the appearance of :
A. Koplik's spots
B. Owl's eye inclusions
C. Heterophile antibodies
D. Cowdry type A inclusions

42. Almost all patients with a lung abscess present with
A. Diarrhea
B. Malaise
C. Cough and fever
D. Weight loss

43. Which of the following statements describes the herpes viruses?
A. Large-sized enveloped viruses with an icosahedral nucleocapsid containing circular, single-stranded DNA.
B. Medium sized enveloped viruses with an icosahedral nucleocapsid containing linear double-stranded RNA.
C. Small-sized enveloped viruses with an icosahedral nucleocapsid containing circular, double stranded DNA.

D. Medium-sized enveloped viruses with an icosahedral nucleocapsid containing linear double-stranded DNA.

44. Which herpes simplex virus listed below causes acute herpetic gingivostomatitis, recurrent herpes labialis, cancre sores, keratoconjunctivitis and encephalitis?

A. Herpes simplex virus type 1 (HSV – 1)
B. Herpes simplex virus type 2 (HSV – 2)
C. Epstein Barr virus
D. None of the above

45. Which of the following is a constituent of gram-negative microorganisms and has been suggested as an important agent in the pathogenesis of inflammatory periodontal disease?

A. Carbohydrates
B. Lipids
C. Exotoxin
D. Endotoxin

46. All of the following statements concerning Respiratory Synctial Virus (RSV) are true, except:

A. It belongs to the orthomyxovirus family
B. Its surface spikes are fusion proteins, not hemagglutinins or neuraminidases.
C. It is the most important cause of severe pneumonia and bronchiolitis in infants.
D. Transmission occurs via respiratory droplets and by direct contact of contaminated hands with the nose or mouth

47. Reoviruses:

A. Have a unique single-shelled capsid that contains a non-segmented double stranded DNA genome.
B. Have a unique double-shelled capsid that contains a segmented single stranded RNA genome
C. Have a unique double-shelled capsid that contains a segmented double stranded RNA genome.
D. Have a unique single-shelled capsid that contains a segmented Single stranded DNA genome.

48. Which bacteria listed below has a THICK murein layer that makes up the cell wall?

A. Gram-positive bacteria
B. Gram-negative bacteria
C. Both of the above
D. None of the above

49. Esophageal varices are the result of which of the following?

A. Kidney stones
B. Portal hypertension
C. Ulcers
D. Diverticulosis

50. Which of the following organs undergoes regeneration?

A. Heart
B. Brain
C. Kidney
D. Liver

51. Which of the following describes the lytic reproduction cycle that releases a large number of phage simultaneously?

A. Two-step growth curve
B. One-step growth curve
C. Horizontal growth curve
D. None of the above

52. Which of the following is the term used to describe the synthesis of mRNA, rRNA, and tRNA from a DNA template?

A. Translation
B. Transcription
C. Transduction
D. Transversion

53. All of the following are benign neoplasms except?

A. Adenoma
B. Fibroma
C. Fibrocarcinoma
D. Hemangioma
E. Lipoma

54. A tumor of striated muscle that may occur in the uterus, vagina, pharynx, and tongue is called what?
A. Fibroma
B. Leiomyoma
C. Rhabdomyoma
D. Lipoma

55. Which of the following types of skin cancer is the most common?
A. Squamous cell carcinoma
B. Basal cell carcinoma
C. Malignant melanoma
D. Oat cell carcinoma

56. Endotoxins are the lipopolysaccharide of the cell wall of which bacteria?
A. Gram-positive bacteria
B. Gram-negative bacteria
C. Fungi
D. Viruses

57. Which of the following induces or forms toxic free—radicals, which cause chemical reactions disruptive to the biochemical organization of microorganisms?
A. Ultraviolet light
B. Ionizing radiation
C. Disinfectants
D. Autoclaving

58. Which of the following bacteria are gram-negative, facultatively anaerobic-rods, motile by means of peritrichous or polar flagella, and divided into five tribes?
A. Enterobacteria
B. Mycobacterium
C. Neisseria
D. Bacteroides

59. Which of the following bacteria form unusual acids, called mycolic acids, that are associated with their cell walls?
A. Escherichia coli
B. Lactobacillus casei

C. Mycobacterium tuberculosis
D. Streptococci

60. Which of the following viruses have spikes that are involved in the absorption of the virus to the host cell?
A. Papovaviruses
B. Adenoviruses
C. Iridoviruses
D. Poxvirus

61. The coxsackie virus is classified under which family name?
A. Togaviridae
B. Orthomyxoviridae
C. Picornaviridae
D. Retroviridae

62. Which virus below is known for its antigenic shift?
A. Rubeola
B. Rubella
C. Influenza
D. Mumps

63. Which of the following is a highly contagious infection of the respiratory tract caused by a myxovirus and transmitted by airborne droplet infection?
A. Anthrax
B. Influenza
C. Gas gangrene
D. Hepatitis B

64. A fetus with the following triad of complications i.e. Cataracts, Cardiac malformations, Deafness probably was infected with what virus?
A. Rubella
B. Herpes simplex
C. Herpes zoster
D. EB virus

65. Which form of hepatitis is characterized by rapid onset of acute signs and symptoms?
A. Hepatitis B

B. Hepatitis A
C. Non A non B
D. Hepatitis D

66. Which group of viruses listed below is frequently found as the causative agent of gastroenteritis?
A. Coxsackie virus
B. Epstein-Barr virus
C. ECHO virus
D. Herpes simplex

67. Which of the following disorders displays the characteristic "Butterfly" rash?
A. Rheumatoid arthritis
B. Systemic lupus erythematosus
C. Myasthenia gravis
D. None of the above

68. Which syndrome below is characterized by multiple intestinal polyps and abnormal mucocutaneous pigmentation, usually over the lips and buccal mucosa?
A. Sjogren's syndrome
B. Peutz-Jeghers syndrome
C. Stevens-Johnson syndrome
D. All of the above

69. Which drug listed below is the drug of choice for treatment of trichomoniasis?
A. Penicillin
B. Metronidazole
C. Nystatin
D. Amphotericin B

70. The drug of choice in treating Candidiasis is which of the following?
A. Penicillin
B. Erythromycin
C. Nystatin
D. Chloramphenicol

71. A group of diverse, widespread unicellular and multicellular eukaryotic organisms, lacking chlorophyll and usually bearing spores and often filaments are what?

A. Bacteria
B. Viruses
C. Fungi
D. All of the above

72. Which genus of fungi listed below infects skin, hair, and nails?

A. Blastomyces
B. Trichophyton
C. Histoplasma
D. Coccidioides

73. Which two protozoans listed below are found in the oral cavity?

A. Giardia
B. Entamoeba
C. Plasmodium
D. Trichomonas

74. Which of the following fungal diseases is seen primarily in patients with chronic debilitating, especially uncontrolled diabetes mellitus?

A. Actinomycosis
B. Histoplasmosis
C. Zygomycosis / mucormycosis
D. Coccidioidomycosis

75. Which of the following is a genus of fungi that is a common contaminant in the laboratory and a cause of nosocomial infections?

A. Blastomyces
B. Coccidiodies
C. Aspergillus
D. None of the above

76. Which of the following is an infectious disease caused by a yeast-like fungus that usually affects only the skin but may invade the lungs, kidneys, central nervous system, and bones?

A. Histoplasmosis

B. Blastomycosis
C. Candidiasis
D. None of the above

77. Which of the following is referred to as valley fever or San Joaquin fever?
A. Coccidioidomycosis
B. Actinomycosis
C. Blastomycosis
D. Mucormycosis

78. All of the following antibiotics are classified as cell-wall inhibitors except?
A. Penicillins
B. Tetracylines
C. Cephalosporins
D. Vancomycin
E. Bacitracin
F. Chloramphenicol
G. Cycloserine

79. Which of the following antibiotics is considered a broad-spectrum antibiotic?
A. Penicillin
B. Cephalosporins
C. Ampicillin
D. Amoxicillin

80. The antibiotic of choice for prophylactic therapy covering dental procedures in a patient with a heart valve abnormality is which of the following?
A. Tetracycline
B. Amoxicillin
C. Erythromycin
D. Lincomycin

81. Aplastic anemia is a sign of toxicity for which antibiotic listed below
A. Pencillin
B. Clindamycin

C. Chloramphenicol
D. Carbencillin

82. Which antibiotic listed below is most efficient in treating infection due to Bacteroides and fusobacterium species?
A. Penicillin
B. Erythromycin
C. Clindamycin
D. Tetracycline

83. The use of vaccines for preventing clinical symptoms after introduction of the virus is most likely to be effective against which two viruses listed below?
A. Influenza
B. Herpes Zoster
C. Rabies
D. Clostridium tetani
E. Rhinoviruses

84. Which class of anti bodies provides the defense against environmental antigens?
A. IgA
B. IgD
C. IgE
D. IgG
E. IgM

85. An injection of a drug into a patient who is allergic to this drug may lead to death due to which of the following
A. Low levels of histamines
B. Anaphylactic shock
C. Hyperglobulinemia
D. Cardiogenic shock

86. Which two antibiotics are usually prescribed in the treatment of rickettsial diseases?
A. Lincomycin
B. Polymyxin B
C. Tetracycline
D. Chloramphenicol

87. An increase in the size of a cell or a group of cells is called what

A. Atrophy
B. Hypertrophy
C. Hyperplasia
D. Dysplasia

88. Cells of which of the following do not have the ability to retain a latent capacity for mitotic division

A. Blood
B. Bone marrow
C. Liver
D. Neurons in the brain

89. A person with the following clinical signs is probably in what physiological state?

A. Reduced cardiac output
B. Circulatory insufficiency
C. Tachycardia
D. Hypotension
E. Pallor and restlessness
F. Diminished urinary output

90. Which type of chronic inflammation is highly cellular and destructive?

A. Granulomatous
B. Banal
C. Agranulomatous
D. All of the above

91. A slowly developing localized thickening of the outer layers of the skin as a result of chronic excessive exposure to the sun is called what?

A. Actinic keratosis
B. Verruca vulgaris
C. Seborrheic keratosis
D. Squamous cell carcinoma
E. None of the above

92. Which of the following is most commonly found in the ovaries or testes

A. An adenoma
B. A teratoma
C. A sarcoma
D. A lipoma

93. Which of the following types of skin cancer most often arises from keratinocytes in the epidermis of elderly individuals who have been excessively exposed to the sun?

A. Malignant melanoma
B. Squamous cell carcinoma
C. Basal cell carcinoma
D. Ameloblastoma

94. The most common place for malignancy of the GI tract to occur is where

A. Stomach
B. Colon
C. Esophagus
D. Anus

95. Neolithic cells characteristically resemble prickle cells and form keratin pearls on the surface of lesions in which of the following

A. Adenocarcinoma
B. Squamous cell carcinoma
C. Basal cell carcinoma
D. Malignant melanoma

96. Which of the following types of skin cancer is considered to be the most severe?

A. Basal cell carcinoma
B. Squamous cell carcinoma
C. Malignant melanoma
D. All of the above

97. Which of the following is the most common malignancy in women?

A. Breast cancer
B. Lung cancer

C. Brain cancer
D. Colon cancer

98. A patient with a painless enlarged lymph node or nodes in the neck who complains of weakness, fever and weight loss is probably suffering from what?
A. Legionnaire's Disease
B. Tay Sach Disease
C. Malignant Lymphoma
D. Leukoplakia

99. Any of several bleeding disorders characterized by hemorrhage into the tissues particularly beneath the skin or mucous membrane, which then produces ecchymoses or petechiae is called what?
A. Purpura
B. Hemophilia
C. Aplastic anemia
D. Agranulocytosis

100. Productive cough, often with wheezing, is universal factor of which disease?
A. Emphysema
B. Lung cancer
C. Chronic bronchitis
D. Asthma

Answer Key to MCQs in Microbiology and Pathology Part III

1	B	2	C	3	B	4	C
5	B	6	B	7	D	8	C
9	C	10	B	11	C	12	B
13	B	14	C	15	C	16	C
17	C	18	G	19	A	20	D
21	F	22	A	23	E	24	C
25	A, D	26	D	27	A	28	D
29	C	30	E	31	A	32	C
33	C	34	D	35	C	36	C
37	C	38	C	39	B	40	C
41	C	42	C	43	D	44	A
45	D	46	A	47	C	48	A
49	B	50	D	51	B	52	B
53	C	54	C	55	B	56	B
57	B	58	A	59	C	60	B
61	C	62	C	63	B	64	A
65	B	66	C	67	B	68	B
69	B	70	C	71	C	72	B
73	B, D	74	C	75	C	76	B
77	A	78	B, F	79	B	80	B
81	C	82	C	83	C, D	84	C
85	B	86	C, D	87	B	88	D
89	Shock	90	A	91	A	92	B
93	B	94	B	95	B	96	C
97	A	98	C	99	A	100	C

Part IV

1. **Which of the following is defined as the accumulation of extravascular fluid in lung tissues and alveoli caused most commonly by congestive heart failure**
   A. Bronchiectasis
   B. Pulmonary emboli
   C. Pulmonary edema
   D. Atelectasis

2. **Which of the following is a closed sac in or under the skin lined with epithelium and containing fluid semisolid material?**
   A. A granuloma
   B. A cyst
   C. An abscess
   D. All of the above

3. **Which of the following bacteria are often responsible for lung abscess?**
   A. Clostridium
   B. Staphylococcus
   C. Bacillus .
   D. Streptococcus

4. **Which bacteria listed below produces the enzyme collagenase?**
   A. Streptococcus pyogenes
   B. Clostridium perfringens
   C. Staphylococcus aureus
   D. Streptococcal sanguis

5. **Which bacteria listed below has been found predominately in cases of advanced periodontitis?**
   A. Bacillus anthracis
   B. Bacteroids melaninogenicus
   C. Streptococcus
   D. Veillonella alcalescens

6. **Which of the following bacteria are notable for their fluorescent pigments and their resistance to disinfectants and antibiotics**
   A. Bacteroides
   B. Pseudomonas
   C. Staphylococci
   D. Treponema

7. **Which of the following bacteria produces a toxin that can be detected using the ELISA assays?**
   A. Bacteroides
   B. E. coli
   C. Neisseria
   D. Eikenella

8. **Which of the following bacteria is the most common cause of urinary tract infection?**
   A. Staphylococcus
   B. Bacteroides
   C. Escherichia
   D. Streptococcus

9. **Organisms belonging to which of the following genera can tolerate the lowest pH?**
   A. Proteus
   B. Clostridium
   C. Lactobacillus
   D. Pseudomonas

10. **Which of the following is a group of gram-positive, asporogenic, regularly shaped rods that produce lactic acid as a major fermentation product?**
    A. Bacteroides
    B. Neisseria
    C. Lactobacillus
    D. Salmonella

11. **Which of the following is a genus of nonmotile, spherical, gram-positive bacteria which may cause severe, purulent**

infections or produce an enterotoxin, which may cause nausea, vomiting and diarrhea?
A. Streptococcus
B. Staphylococcus
C. Neisseria
D. Salmonella

12. Which virus listed below can cause herpes zoster lesions along sensory nerve roots in later life?
A. Poxvirus
B. Epstein-Barr virus
C. Varicella virus
D. HSV I virus

13. An infection or inflammation of the membranes covering the brain and spinal cord is called what?
A. Meningitis
B. Encephalitis
C. Meningism
D. None of the above

14. Cytopathic effects (CPE) are due to infection by which of the following?
A. Fungi
B. Viruses
C. Spirochetes
D. All of the above

15. Which of the following species is known to produce the enzyme penicillinase?
A. Streptococcus
B. Bacillus
C. Neisseria
D. Staphylococcus

16. The erythrogenic toxin produced by streptococcus pyogenes causes which disease?
A. Gas gangrene
B. Bacterial dysentery
C. Scarlet fever
D. Tetanus

17. Dental caries is initiated at the tooth surface as a result of the growth of which species listed below?

A. Staphylococcus
B. Pseudomonas
C. Streptococcus
D. Bacteroides

18. Which two bacteria listed below are referred to as lactic acid bacteria?

A. Streptococcus
B. Lactobacillus
C. Staphylococcus
D. Bacteroids

19. What two bacteria listed below cause impetigo?

A. Streptococcus
B. Neisseria
C. Staphylococcus
D. Bacteroides

20. Which bacteria listed below is penicillin-resistant?

A. Streptococcus pyogenes
B. Streptococcus fecalis
C. Streptococcus pneumoniae
D. None of the above

21. The majority of bacterial pneumonias are caused by which etiologic agent listed below?

A. Streptococcus
B. Klebsiella
C. Haemophilus influenza
D. Clostridium

22. Chemical agents that kill microorganisms are called what?

A. Germicides
B. Microbiostatic agents
C. Disinfectants
D. Antiseptics

23. IgE is involved in which of the four types of hypersensitivity reactions?

A. Type 1
B. Type 2
C. Type 3
D. Type 4

24. All of the following diseases are classified as what?

A. Serum sickness
B. Systemic lupus-erythematosus
C. Glomerulonephritis
D. Autoimmune hemolysis
E. Rheumatoid arthritis

Answer = immune complex diseases

25. Which of the following is a mixture of leukotrienes that acts as a potent bronchial constrictor?

A. Heparin
B. Histamine
C. Slow-reacting substance of anaphylaxis
D. Dopamine

26. Which of the following cell types is found in great abundance at the inflamed site?

A. Macrophages
B. Basophils
C. Eosinophils
D. Neutrophils

27. Which of the following is the principal chemical mediator located in the granules of mast cells and basophils?

A. Bradykinin
B. Plasmin
C. Histamine
D. Complement

28. Which of the following refers to a disease or microorganism that is indigenous to a geographic area or population?

A. Endemic
B. Pandemic

C. Epidemic
D. Epizootic

29. Which of the following is defined as a modified protein exotoxin that has lost its toxicity but has retained its specific antigenicity?
A. Antitoxin
B. Toxoid
C. Hapten
D. None

30. The enzyme catalase is contained in which organelle within a cell?
A. Nucleus
B. Microbodies
C. Golgi apparatus
D. Lysosomes

31. Which of the following is a nonproteinaceous substance that acts as antigen by combining with particular bonding sites on an antibody?
A. Lipids
B. Plasmids
C. Haptens
D. Flagella

32. Which of the following is an interactive association between two populations of different species living together in which one population benefits from the association , while the other is not affected?
A. Symbiosis
B. Mutualism
C. Commensalisms
D. Latency

33. A chronic infectious disease of the eye characterized by inflammation, pain, photophobia, and lacrimation is called what?
A. Pink eye
B. Trachoma
C. Inclusion conjunctivitis

34. Urethritis, dysuria, purulent, greenish-yellow urethral or vaginal discharge, red or oedematous meatus, and itching, burning, or pain around the vagina or urethral orifice are characteristic of which disease?

A. Syphilis
B. Gonorrhea
C. Herpes
D. HIV

35. Primary syphilis produces which of the following on the genitalia?

A. Rash
B. Chancre
C. Bruise
D. Gummas

36. Anthrax, botulism, gas gangrene, and tetanus are caused by which type of bacteria?

A. Spore-forming
B. Nonspore-forming
C. Fungi
D. Viruses

37. Which of the following statements describes the herpes viruses?

A. Large-sized viruses containing circular, single-stranded DNA
B. Medium-sized viruses containing linear, double-stranded DNA
C. Small-sized viruses containing circular, double-stranded DNA
D. Small-sized viruses containing circular, single-stranded RNA

38. The common cold, influenza, measles, mumps, chicken pox and infections mononucleosis are all caused by which type of pathogen ?

A. Viral
B. Bacteria
C. Fungal
D. Rickettsial

39. Short term immunity brought about by the transfer of preformed antibody from an immune subject to a non - immune subject is called what

A. Autoimmunity
B. Passive immunity
C. Hypersensitivity
D. Natural Immunity

40. Leukocytes often accompany which type of infection?

A. Viral
B. Bacterial
C. Fungal
D. Parasitic

41. The following biochemical mediators are called what?

A. Macrophage chemotactic factor
B. Migration inhibitory factor
C. Interlukin-1
D. Interlacing - 2
E. Platelet activating factor
Answer = lymphokines

42. The following elements make up what system?

A. Macrophages
B. Kupffer cells of the liver
C. Reticulum cells of lungs
D. Bone marrow
E. Lymph nodes and spleen
Answer = reticuloendothelial system

43. Which of the following is an abnormal condition in which the kidneys are enlarged and contain many sacs

A. Glomerulonephritis
B. Polycystic kidney
C. Secondary amyloidosis
D. All of the above

44. Which of the following is a progressive megaloblastic, macrocytic anemia affecting mainly older people ?

A. Thalassemia major
B. Thalassemia minor

C. Pernicious anemia
D. Aplastic anemia

45. Which of the following types of hemophilia is also called the Christmas diseases?
A. Hemophilia - A
B. Hemophilia B
C. Hemophilia C
D. None of the above

46. A patient taking dicumarol can be expected to have which of the following ?
A. Normal blood clotting
B. Delayed blood clotting
C. Enhanced blood clotting

47. Which of the following is an aggregation of blood platelets, fibrin, clotting factor and cellular elements that forms in the heart in the process of dying?
A. Mural thrombus
B. Agonal thrombus
C. White thrombus
D. Red thrombus

48. Which of the following is a naturally occurring derivative of tryptophan found in platelets and in cells of the brain and the intestine
A. Histamine
B. Bradykinin
C. Serotonin
D. Plasma

49. Which blood group listed below has agglutinins neither A or B?
A. A
B. B
C. O
D. AB

50. Which 2 enzymes of the following are elevated in a patient suffering from acute pancreatitis?
A. Alkaline phosphatase

B. Acid phosphatase
C. Lipase
D. Amylase

51. Which of the following complications of peptic ulcers is the most infrequent and accounts for nearly two thirds of all deaths in peptic ulcer patients?
A. Hemorrhage
B. Obstruction of the GI tract from edema scars
C. Perforation
D. Atresia

52. Vomiting of bright red blood indicating rapid upper gastrointestinal bleeding is called what ?
A. Hematomyelia
B. Hematuria
C. Hematemesis
D. Hemosiderosis

53. The most likely diagnosis for a patient with hemoptyses, pain in the chest, weight loss, anorexia, nausea, vomiting and a history of heavy smoking is what ?
A. Carcinoma of the larynx
B. Laryngeal polyps
C. Carcinoma of the lungs
D. Basal cell carcinoma

54. Which of the following is the fragmentation of chromatin filaments and distribution of it through the cytoplasm as result of nuclear disintegration?
A. Karyopyknosis
B. Pyknosis
C. Karyolysis
D. Karyorrhexis

55. A patient with the following symptom is probably suffering from what disorder?
A. Polyuria
B. Polydipsia
C. Hyperglycemia
D. Glycosuria

E. Weight loss
F. Polyphagia
Answer = diabetes mellitus

56. Which of the following is described as the deposition of calcium salt in previously undamaged tissues?
A. Dystrophic calcification
B. Metastatic calcification
C. Calcinosis
D. Tophi

57. Which of the following is the most common form of cancer in men over the age of 50 aside from skin cancer ?
A. Lung
B. Prostate
C. Liver
D. Bone

58. Which of the following is a severe infection of one or more of the five major lobes of the lungs which if untreated eventually result in consolidation of lung tissue?
A. Bronchopneumonia
B. Emphysema
C. Lobar Pneumonia
D. Asthma

59. A chronic lung disease that results in the development of alveolar, interstitial and pleural fibrosis is called as:
A. Anthracosis
B. Asbestosis
C. Berylliosis
D. Silicosis

60. Burton's congenital agammaglobulinemia results in the failure of which cell to differentiate and produce antibodies?
A. T - cells
B. Macrophage
C. Monocytes
D. B - Cells

61. A sex linked inherited condition characterized by the absence of gamma globulin in the blood is called as?

A. Hodgkin's disease
B. Bruton's agammaglobulinemia
C. Thalassemia major
D. None of the above

62. Which of the following is a rare & severe illness of unknown cause mostly affecting young males and characterized by severe uveitis and retinal vasculitis?

A. Multiple myeloma
B. Bahcet's disease
C. Rubeola
D. Pernicious anemia

63. Reversible oxidation - reduction carriers in respiration are called as?

A. Pyramidine nucleotides
B. Cytochromes
C. Reductant
D. Surfactants

64. When nitrate or sulfate serves as the terminal electron acceptor, the metabolic pathway is called what

A. Aerobic respiration
B. Anaerobic respiration
C. Fermentation
D. None of the above

65. An increased serum alkaline phosphatase level is clinically significant and aids in the diagnosis of which of the following condition

A. Hyperparathyroidism
B. Paget's disease of bone
C. Prostate carcinoma
D. Hepatitis B

66. Haberden's nodes are diagnostic of which type of arthritis ?

A. Rheumatoid arthritis
B. Osteoarthritis

C. Hyperuricemia
D. None of the above

67. Anemia, hemorrhage, splenomegaly, lymphadenopathy, and localized tumefactions over bones are usually present in which disease
A. Multiple myeloma
B. Lettere Siwe disease
C. Hand Schuller Christian disease
D. Osteoradionecrosis

68. A patient with increased bone density / marble bone, hydrocephalus, blindness, deafness, dental caries and facial palsies is most likely suffering from what
A. Osteopetrosis
B. Osteogenesis imperfecta
C. Achondroplasia
D. Fibrous dysplasia

69. A malignant tumor developing from bone marrow, usually in long bones or the pelvis of adolescent boys is called what?
A. Myeloma
B. Ewing's sarcoma
C. Osteogenic sarcoma
D. Squamous cell carcinoma

70. Which of the following is the physiological function of Vitamin A?
A. Hemopoiesis
B. Collagen formation
C. Production of rhodopsin
D. Absorption of calcium

71. Which of the following vitamins functions in collagen formation?
A. B
B. C
C. D
D. A

72. The Philadelphia chromosome is present in myeloblasts in most patients with which disease listed below?
A. Multiple myeloma
B. Chronic myelocytic leukemia
C. Aplastic anemia
D. Gaucher's disease

73. There is no conclusive evidence of a causative infectious agent to which disease listed below?
A. Herpes
B. Infectious Mononucleosis
C. Hodgkin's disease
D. Mumps

74. Which of the following is a characteristic of malignancy?
A. Dysplasia
B. Anaplasia
C. Metaplasia
D. Aplasia

75. Which of the following is a malignant, usually bronchogenic epithelial neoplasm consisting of small, tightly packed, round, oval, or spindle-shaped epithelial cells that stain darkly & contain neurosecretory granules and little or no cytoplasm?
A. Adenocarcinoma
B. Squamous cell carcinoma
C. Oat cell carcinoma
D. Basal cell carcinoma

76. Which syndrome listed below is a condition found in males with one or more extra X chromosomes?
A. Klinefelter's syndrome
B. Turner 's syndrome
C. Down's syndrome
D. None of the above

77. Secondary hyperparathyroidism results from which of the following?
A. Adenoma
B. Hypertension

C. Chronic renal disease
D. Diabetes

78. Name the condition that is associated with hypertension in which there is necrosis of the renal arterioles.
A. Acute nephritis
B. Nephrosclerosis
C. Chronic pyelonephritis
D. Nephrosis

79. Which of the following lesions is most common in the adrenal medulla of young children?
A. Malignant melanoma
B. Basal cell carcinoma
C. Neuroblastoma
D. Squamous cell carcinoma

80. Renal calculi occur in approximately 75 percent of all patients with which disorder?
A. Polycystic kidney
B. Glomerulonephritis
C. Hyperparathyroidism
D. Hypoparathyroidism

81. Which two glands listed below fail to develop in children with the DiGeorge syndrome?
A. Thyroid
B. Adrenal
C. Thymus
D. Pituitary
E. Parathyroid

82. Compression of the heart produced by the accumulation in the pericardial sac of fluid or of blood resulting from the rupture of a blood vessel of the myocardium is called what?
A. Constrictive pericarditis
B. Mitral stenosis
C. Cardiac tamponade
D. Hypertension

83. Which three organs below get damaged by prolonged hypertension?

A. Heart
B. Intestine
C. Brain
D. Stomach
E. Kidneys

84. Tissue from another species used as a temporary graft in certain cases, as in treating a severely burned patient, is called what?

A. Xenograft
B. Autograft
C. Allograft
D. Isograft

85. Which healing process of a wound listed below would contain granulation tissue?

A. First intention
B. Second intention

86. A chronic metabolic condition characterized by a gradual, marked enlargement and elongation of the bones of the face, jaw, and extremities afflicting middle-aged adults is called what?

A. Acromegaly
B. Gigantism
C. Cretinism
D. None of the above

87. Which of the following is a proteolytic enzyme, produced by & stored in the juxtaglomerular apparatus that surrounds each arteriole as it enters a glomerulus?

A. Plasmin
B. Lysozyme
C. Renin
D. Pepsin

88. The acid fast stain may be performed on many clinical specimens but is most commonly used in examining sputum for which bacteria listed below

A. Escherichia coli
B. Streptococcus pneumonia
C. Clostridium botulinum
D. Mycobacterium tuberculosis

Answer Key to MCQs in Microbiology and Pathology Part IV

1	C	2	B	3	B	4	B
5	B	6	B	7	B	8	C
9	C	10	C	11	B	12	C
13	A	14	B	15	D	16	C
17	C	18	A, B	19	A, C	20	B
21	A	22	A	23	A	24	=
25	C	26	D	27	C	28	A
29	B	30	B	31	C	32	C
33	B	34	B	35	B	36	A
37	B	38	A	39	B	40	B
41	=	42	=	43	B	44	C
45	B	46	B	47	B	48	C
49	D	50	C, D	51	C	52	C
53	C	54	D	55	=	56	B
57	B	58	C	59	B	60	D
61	B	62	B	63	B	64	B
65	B	66	B	67	B	68	A
69	B	70	C	71	B	72	B
73	C	74	B	75	C	76	A
77	C	78	B	79	C	80	C
81	C, E	82	C	83	A,C,E	84	A
85	B	86	A	87	C	88	D

15

Pharmacology

ANALGESICS

- Most **analgesics will have no perceptible effects on acute pulpitis**, PDL or periapical abscess if physical measures are not taken by the dentist to actively relieve the pain, drainage.
- **Aspirin is C/I in children as it can cause Reye's syndrome,** i.e. a fatty degeneration in liver and kidney with an associated encephalopathy with high morbidity and mortality.
- Anticoagulant action of coumarin type drugs e.g. warfarin is enhanced by aspirin.
- Aspirin increase acid production in GIT, while prostaglandins exert protective action on GIT by decreasing acid production.
- Aspirin has **antidiabetic action** by increasing peripheral use of glucose.
- **Opioids should not be given** to patients with a suspected **head injury** as the drug may mask pupillary evidence of increasing intracranial pressure by its effect on the pupillo-constrictor centers.
- **Carbamazepine** = used in Rx of epilepsy but also for Rx of **trigeminal neuralgia**. It is not an analgesic but it is a membrane-stabilising agent.
- **Antibiotic** = is a substance which cause the death of or prevents successful replication of microbes.
- A **bactericidal** agent = drug kill the sensitive organisms.
- **Bacteriostatic** agent = which prevent the successful reproduction.

- In general, a bactericidal + bactericidal agent = synergistic effect,
- But, a bactericidal + bacteriostatic agent = antagonism effect. THIS combination **should be avoided** because bacteriostatic agents interfere with multiplication / reproduction of microbes, while for the successful action of bactericidal agents, a multiplying organism is required.
- Narrow spectrum antibiotics = have limited range of effect, normally vs G + bacteria.
- Broad spectrum antibiotics = have activity vs G +, G – bacteria and sometimes mycoplasma.
- Use of combined antibiotic Rx should be reserved for severe infections.
- **Anxiolytic** drugs = which reduce anxiety, tension or fear.
- **Hypnotics** = which induce sleep.
- Mechanism of action of *benzodiazepines* = bind to GABA receptors mainly in cerebral cortex and augment the GABA activity.

LOCAL ANAESTHESIA

Components of local anaesthesia

1.	2% lignocaine–HCl:	21.3 mg.	Main component
2.	Adrenaline	0.005 mg	vasoconstrictor
3.	Sodium chloride	6.0 mg	isotonicity of solution
4.	Sodium metabisulphite	0.5 mg	preservative of adrenaline.
5.	Methyl paraben	1.0 mg	preservative/ fungicide
6.	Water to make	1.0 ml	vehicle

Block	Teeth involved
Inferior dental block	All lower teeth
Mental nerve block	Lower first PM to CI
Infraorbital nerve	Upper CI to PM2.
Nasopalatine block	Mucoperiosteum palatal to upper incisors and canines
Greater palatine block	Mucoperiosteum palatal to upper PMs and molars.
Posterior superior alveolar block	Upper molars
Lingual nerve block	Ant 2/3rd tongue, floor of mouth and lingual gingiva

Important

Ester group	Mainly metabolised by **plasma cholinesterase;** some in liver
Amide group	Metabolised only **in liver**
Prilocaine	Metabolised **in lungs also**
Procaine	Metabolised **in kidneys also**
Chloroprocaine	**Least toxic; safest;** used in children; short acting
Tetracaine	**Most toxic;** compatible with sulfonamides; only topical use
Cocaine	Only LA with **vasoconstrictor** property; excreted unaltered by kidneys so C/I in kidneys disease; used only topically.
Procaine	First synthetic LA; **greatest vasodilating** property of all LA.
Propoxycaine	Always combined with 2 % procaine; useful **in absolute C/I of amide** type LA.

Importants (*Contd.*)

Propoxycaine/ rovacaine	Effective in **inflammed tissues**
Lidocaine	**First non- ester** type of LA; suitable in inflammed tissues; agent of choice in patients with abnormal amounts of plasma cholinesterase enzyme
Mepivacaine	Longer duration; can be used in patients where **Adr is not recommended** (hyperthyroidism)
Priolocaine	May cause **methemoglobulinemia**
Prilocaine + 1: 2 lac Adr	Safest amide LA; **longest** duration effect
Bupivacaine	Long acting; no need of post – op. Analgesics; should not be given in children
Articaine	Metabolised by **saponification**/ hydrolysis in liver; only LA C/I in patients allergic to Sulphur containing compounds
Etidocaine	Not given in children due to longer duration; rapid redistribution
Amide LA	C/I in patients with **malignant hyperthermia**
Benzocaine	Topical; inhibits sulfonamides
Dyclonine HCl	Given in patients with **known sensitivity** to LAs
Centbucridine	No CNS/ CVS effects
Allergy	Common with ester type LA; due to PABA, methyl paraben
Toxicity of LA	First S/S is CNS effects is TALKATIVENESS

- **Ester group** local anaesthesia is metabolised by **plasma cholinestrase** and some in liver; **Amide type** local anaesthesia **in liver only** by microsomal enzymes.

- **Prilocaine** in small % is metabolised **in lungs** also.
- **Procaine** also undergoes some biotransformation in **kidney.**
- **Ester type local anaesthesia should not be given in the patients with cholinesterase deficiency , but amide type can be used.**
- Local anaesthesia = **prilocaine is biotransformed in = lungs**; all others are biotransformed in liver.
- **Cocaine is excreted unchanged**; all others are excreted via urine.
- Except cocaine, all LA are vasodilators.
- Prilocaine produces = **methemoglobulinemia** by orthotoluidine
- Propoxycaine = LA **effective in inflammed** tissues.
- Mepivacaine = has **negligible topical activity**, low pka; used in pus, **indicated in hyperthyroid;** C/I in renal disease.
- Bupivacaine, etidocaine = **longest duration of action**
- A resting nerve is more resistant to blockade compared to conducting nerve.
- LA enters the axon at the **node of Ranvier only**.
- Autonomic fibres are more susceptible to blockade than a somatic fibre.
- LA are **cardiac depressant**.
- Chlorprocaine is a rapid onset LA despite having a high pka.
- LA with Vasoconstrictor should not be injected for ring blocks of hands, feet, fingers, toes etc. due to risk of gangrene.
- Only indication of cocaine now- a- days is **ocular anaesthesia**.
- For **spinal anaesthesia**, LA is injected in the subarachnoid space b/w L 2-3 or 3- 4 level , i.e. below the lower end of spinal cord.

Important Points based on MCQs:

- APC = aspirin + phenacetin + caffeine
- Penicillinase resistance gonococci respond to = spectinomycin
- G + BACTERIA ARE MORE SENSITIVE TO PENICILLINS than G – bacteria = due to **cell wall** composition. G + bacteria have **peptidoglycans,** whose cross-linking is prevented by

penicillin, so rigid cell wall is not formed. G – bacteria have lipopolysaccharides in cell wall.

- Most effective antibacterial agents are = cationic.
- Actinomyces group supplies largest no. of antibiotics.
- Sporulating bacteria produce = polypeptide antibiotics.
- Sporulating fungi produce = penicillins and cephalosporins.
- Penicillins require growing bacteria for its action, but any bacteriostatic agents interfere with this.
- **Lente-insulin** = crystalline : amorphous insulin in 7:3.
- **Procaine penicillin fortified** = procaine penicillin : sodium penicillin in 3:1.
- Sulfonamide : trimethoprim = 5:1.
- Ampicillin has best G (-) spectrum among penicillins.
- **Clindamycin** = given in prophylaxis of SABE if patient is allergic to penicillin and erythromycin.
- Antihistaminics = increase the no. of MACROPHAGES.
- Astemizol, an Antihistaminics = longest duration of action.
- **Heparin** interferes with clot formation by = preventing thrombin formation from prothrombin (**anti-thrombin** action), i.e. **second-last step**.
- Heparin prevents = **arterial clotting** disorders
- Coumarine etc. prevent = **venous clotting** disorders
- Among tetracyclines = **only doxycycline** is excreted by liver, all others are excreted in urine.
- Tetracycline **blocks the activity of collagenase** so helpful in periodontitis.
- Penicillinase resistance antibiotic = **methicillin**
- Penicillin = treatment of gonococcal, syphilis, actinomyces, pneumococcal infections
- Tetracycline = in treatment of cholera, rickettsial infections,

- Chloramphenicol = for typhoid.
- INH causes vit B_{12} deficiency.
- Methotrexate causes **folic acid deficiency.**
- Betamethasone is most inflammatory.
- Aldosterone is least inflammatory.

ANTICANCER DRUGS

- Mercaptopurine = decrease purine synthesis
- Methotrexate = folate antagonist
- Alkylating agents = produce carbonium ions
- Antibiotics = interfere with template DNA function
- Cisplastin = radiomimetic action, cause cross-linking of DNA
- Plant alkaloids = mitotic inhibitors, bind to **tubulin** and cause **disruption of mitotic spindles**.
- Levodopa = does not cause sedation
- Phenothiazine = antipsychotic, antiemetic

BENZODIAZEPINES

- Benzodiazepines = GABA facilitatory
- I/V diazepam = **thrombophlebitis** due to **propylene glycol**; it can be overcome by DIAZEMULS.
- Most effective agent to treat respiratory depression due to overdose of barbiturate = oxygen.
- Barbiturates = GABA facilitatory and GABA mimetic.
- Promethazine/phenargen = it is phenothiazine, but not antipsychotic, it is **antihistaminic**, so used in parkinsonism developed after injection of **prochlorprazine** which is also a phenothiazine.
- Sudden withdrawal of phenobarbitone precipitates = status epilepticus.
- Phenobarbitone = is not preferred in temporal lobe epilepsy.

ANTIHYPERTENSIVE

- Combination necessary to block the CVS effects produced by injection of sympathomimetic drugs are = prazosine + propranolol (alpha, beta-blocker)
- **Propranolol** = is a cardiac depressant ; is of value in angina because it **prevents chronotropic response** to endogenous epinephrine, emotions, exercise.
- Propranolol is **C/I in** = cardiac arrhythmia, hypoglycemia, partial or complete heart block, asthma, in p.o. adr., CHF, AV-block.
- Propranolol is a beta 1 and beta 2 acting and **without intrinsic sympathomimetic** activity drug.
- Which drug decreases BP by **activating alpha –2 receptors** in medulla (VMC) = clonidine
- Methoxamine = for increasing BP, without cardiac stimulation but by **increase in peripheral resistance.**
- **Methacholine** = has both negative inotropic and negative chronotropic effects.
- **Hydralazine** = both increased HR and CO.
- Verapamil = for *atrial tachycardia* (V–AT).
- Guanethidine = anti – HT drug, causes exaggerated response to an injected catecholamine.
- Increase in HR due to nitroglycerine is antagonised by propranolol.
- Anti HT drug having **a unique property of** increasing HR and CO = hydralazine.
- **Reserpine** – an antihypertensive agent. It acts at membrane of intra neuronal granules which store monoamines, i.e. NA, 5 – HT; DA and irreversibly inhibits the active transport. It is an HIT and RUN DRUG; it causes Catecholamine and 5 – HT depletion; increases HCl secretion in stomach. It **prevents reuptake of N-Adr by storage granules** in the nerve terminals. Since enz monoamine oxidase is required for metabolism of NA so, in p.o. of MAO – I, there is no metabolism of NA.

- Treatment of Atrial tachycardia and supraventricular tachycardia = verapamil or procainamide
- Treatment of ventricular tachycardia = lignocaine
- Treatment of supraventricular tachyarrhythmia = quinidine
- Treatment of Atrial and ventricular arrhythmia = quinidine and procainamide
- Treatment of Atrial arrhythmia = digitalis
- Treatment of Atrial tachycardia and digitalis induced arrhythmia = propranolol
- Treatment of Ventricular conduction disturbance = lidocaine
- Treatment of Atrial fibrillation = quinidine
- Treatment of Atrial arrhythmia = phenytoin
- Treatment of ventricular arrhythmia = phenytoin
- Treatment of digitalis – induced arrhythmia = phenytoin
- Treatment of Atrial arrhythmia, MI, CHF = digitalis
- Treatment of s/s of hyperthyroidism = by beta-blockers

- Phenytoin = nerve membrane stabilising effect.
- Alcohol use = korsakoft-syndrome
- Tricyclic antidepressants = anticholinergic ANS action, muscarinic blockade
- Atropine = reduces secretions, depresses vagal reflex,
- **Spironolactone** = diuresis is due to a **direct antagonism of aldosterone**.
- Diuretic used in treatment of epilepsy = **acetazolamide**. It is a **carbonic anhydrase inhibitor**, increases CO_2 conc in CNS; acts as adjuvant to its treatment.

Drugs of choice/antidotes

Actinomycosis	Penicillin – G iv
Acute barbiturate poisoning	Pentylene tetrazole
Adrenergically induced arrythmia	Propranolol
Alcohol addiction	Disulfiram
Amoebiasis	Metronidazole
Anaphylactic shock	Adrenaline
Atrial tachycardia	Propranolol
Bezalkonium chloride	Soaps
Burkit's lymphoma	Cyclophosphamide
CML	Busulfan
Copper	EDTA, BAL
Curare	Anticholinesterases
Cyanide poisoning	Sodium nitrate i.v.
d- tubocurarine	Neostigmine
Datura	Physostigmine
Diazepam poisoning	Flumazenil
Gout/chronic gout	Indomethacin/probenecid respectively
Grand mal epilepsy	Phenytoin, phenobarbitone/ barbiturates
Heparin antagonist	Protamine sulphate
Hg – poisoning	Dimercaprol / BAL
Hypertensive emergency	Sod. Nitroprusside, GTN
Increased intracranial pressure	Mannitol i.v.
Iron poisoning	Desferrioxamine

Drugs of choice/antidotes (*Contd.*)

LSD	Tranquilizers
Lymphogranuloma venerum	Tetracycline
Malignant hyperthermia	Dentrolene sodium i.v
Methicillin resistance	Vancomycin
Methotrexate poisoning	Folinic acid
Migraine (prophylaxis)	Propranolol oral
Morphine poisoning	Naloxone
Myasthenia gravis	Neostigmine oral
Obstetric local analgesia	Bupivacaine
Opium	Naloxone HCl
Organophosphate/ anticholinesterase poisoning	Pralidoxime/Atropine i.v.
Pb – poisoning	Sodium calcium edetate
PCM poisoning	N – acetyl cysteine
Penicillinase resistance	Methicillin
Peripheral poisons are	Curare, conium maculatum
Petitmal epilepsy	Ethosuximide/Sod. valproate
Phenoxybenzamine	Epinephrine
Post-partum hemorrhage	Methyl ergotamine
Relapsing fever	Tetracycline
Rheumatic fever	Aspirin
Rheumatoid arthritis	Aspirin
Roundworm infestation	Albendazole
Scopolamine	Physostigmine

Drugs of choice/antidotes (*Contd.*)

Spinal poison is	Strychnine
Status epilepticus and tonic clonic seizures	Diazepam
Syphilis	Benzathine penicillin i.m
Thyrotoxicosis	Carbamazole
Treatment of atropine overdose	Physostigmine
Treatment of d-tubocurarine overdose	Neostigmine
Treatment of neostigmine overdose	Atropine
Trigeminal neuralgia	Carbamazepine
Typhoid/ enteric fever	Ciprofloxacin
Ulcerative colitis	Sulfasalazine oral
Vit B_6	Desoxypyridoxine

Treatment of lymphatic leukemia = chlorambucil

Treatment of myeloid leukemia = busulfan

Treatment of multiple myeloma = malphalan

Antiviral drugs

1. Zidovudine = HIV
2. Amantadine = influenza
3. Acyclovir = herpes group
4. Idoxuridine = HS- I (Herpes Simplex - 1)

Chloroquine

- Drug of choice for all malaria **except due to P. falciparum** and prophylaxis
- Drug of choice for radical cure of malaria = primaquine

- Chloroquine resisted can be controlled by = methoquine
- Chloroquine intolerant malaria = by pyrimethamine
- Doses of chloroquine = 600 mg stat ; 300 mg after 8 hrs ; 300 mg daily for 2 days (total = 1500 mg).

PREGNANCY

- **Antibiotics to be avoided** in it = tetracyclines, aminoglycosides e.g. streptomycin, gentamycin, neomycin etc.; cotrimoxazole, etc.
- Oral contraceptives cause proliferation of subgingival black pigmented bacteroides; its side effect is that it predisposes patient to **thrombophlebitis**.
- **Tetracycline** alters gut flora and **decreases plasma levels of estrogen**, so females taking it may be at an increased risk of pregnancy.
- For rest = supine position should be avoided; **left lateral decubitus position should be used**, so as to avoid pressure on IVC and venous return.
- Penicillin and cephalosporins = are safe in pregnancy
- **Acetaminophen** = **analgesic of choice** in pregnants
- Aspirin = hazards of **intracranial hemorrhage** in premature infants
- Sulfonamides = cause neonatal kernicterus
- Alcohol use during pregnancy = causes fetal alcohol syndrome.
- Fluoride = partially crosses the placenta.
- **Metronidazole** = is mutagenic in I st trimester
- **Lidocaine** = safe
- Clindamycin = causes pseudomembranous colitis
- Gentamycin = ototoxicity
- Erythromycin esteolate = hepatotoxicity
- Diazepam = craniofacial defects
- Morphine sulphate = drug of choice to relieve maternal anxiety
- Folic acid = helps **neural tube development** in fetus.
- Tetracycline = staining of teeth; so avoid it; teratogenic effects.

CPR

- During CPR, respiratory vs cardiac message should be = 1: 5
- Resting tidal volume given must be = 2 × the normal

MECHANISM OF ACTION OF DRUGS

Cycloserine, bacitracin, vancomycin, penicillin	Block **cell wall synthesis** of bacteria
Tetracycline, erythromycin, lincomycin	Inhibit **protein synthesis**
Antifungal antibiotics	**Not active vs bacteria** because bacterial cell wall has no sterols
Sulfa drugs	By inducing **folic acid deficiency** by competing with PABA
Anti arrhythmic	**Increase refractory period** of cardiac muscles
Antihistaminics	Compete with histamine for peripheral receptors
LA	**Prevents depolarisation of nerve membrane** and generation of nerve action potential
Alpha and beta blockers	**Competitive inhibition** of post-junctional adrenergic receptors
Digitalis	**Decreases rate of AV-conduction** and increases force of contraction
Antipsychotic	Dopaminergic blockers e.g. phenothiazines
Spironolactone	**Antagonises aldosterone** and so diuresis occurs

MECHANISM OF ACTION OF DRUGS (*Contd.*)

Alpha- methyl DOPA	Forms a false transmitter, the effect of which is primarily at central nuclei
Nitroglycerine/ GTN	**Dilates coronary A.** by direct action on smooth ms. in vessel wall
Neostigmine	Can directly act on **motor end plates**
Reserpine	**Prevents reuptake of nor-adr** by storage granules in nerve terminals.
Inhaled ammonia	**Irritates the** sensory endings of Vth nerve
Prazosin	**Inhibits postsynaptic action** of nor- adr. On vascular smooth ms.
Morphine	Activates the receptors for the **enkephlins**
Cocaine	Only LA which increases pressor activity of both adr and nor-adr. It also **causes most powerful stimulation** of cerebral cortex.
Central ms relaxants	Depress polysynaptic reflex arcs
Atropine/ scopolamine	**Compete with Ach** for receptors site
Diazepams	Act by modulating GABA
Sulphonyl urea, i.e. oral hypoglycemics	By stimulating pancreatic secretion of insulins
LA aids in	Decreasing salivary flow by reducing sensitivity and anxiety during tooth preparation.
MAOI	By noncompetitive inhibition
Propranolol	**Anti-renin** effect
Antidepressants/ imipramine	**Block reuptake of** amine neurotransmitters released into synaptic clefts.

MECHANISM OF ACTION OF DRUGS (*Contd.*)

Guanethidine	Depletes NA from nerve terminals
Captopril	Anti-HT by accumulation of **bradykinin** metabolites.
Anticancer drugs Alkylating agents	Carbonium ions are produced which cause defective base pair formation in DNA formation, thus **DNA synthesis** is impaired.
Antimetabolites	Competitively **inhibit substrate formation** and incorporation into the DNA molecules
Vinca derivatives	**Mitosis inhibitors;** bind to microtubules; inhibit spindle formation and chromosal migration ; ka **metaphase cell arrest.**
Antibiotics	Intercalate b/w DNA macromolecules; rendering it **incapable of decoding** and cell death.
Epipodophyllins	**G_2 phase** of cell cycle is affected.
Hydroxyureas	Inhibit **DNA formation**
Procarbazine	Depolymerizes the DNA molecules thereby damaging the **chromosomal material** of cell and cell death.
Alpha – asparaginase	Cancer cells differ from normal cells in that they lack alpha – asparagine synthetase. This drug deprive the tumor cells of alpha – aspartic acid and so cell death.
Cisplastin	Causes cross linking of DNA macro-molecules, and so inhibit DNA formation.

Pairs having opposite actions

1. Morphine – papavarine
2. Neostigmine – atropine
3. Ach. – Adr.

4. Epinephrine – CPZ (ka **epinephrine reversal of Dale**)
5. Epinephrine – prazosine (for **epinephrine reversal** of BP)
6. Epinephrine antagonises the effects of histamine by producing physiological action opposite to that of histamine.
7. Epinephrine reversal phenomenon is seen with = **alpha-blockers**
8. Phenylepherine = least sympathetic activity but can be used in LA solutions
9. Isoproterenol = cannot be used in LA solution, (no stimulating activity).

Physostigmine = central & peripheral actions Neostigmine = only peripheral actions Levodopa = central & peripheral actions Carbidopa = only peripheral actions

ADRENERGIC RECEPTORS

Receptors	**Location**
Alpha 1	post junctional on effector organs
Alpha 2	prejunctional on nerve endings; post junctional in brain also.
Beta 1	in heart, adipose tissues, JG cells of kidney
Beta 2	Bronchi, blood vessels, uterus

Receptors	**Selective antagonists**	**Selective agonists**
Alpha 1	Prazosine	Phenylephrine
Alpha 2	Yohimbine	Clonidine
Beta 1	Metoprolol	Isoprenalterol
Beta 2	Butoxamine	Salbutamol
	Ie PYMB	Ie PCIS

Isoproterenol / isoprenalin = has **only beta - action;**

Phenylephrine = has alpha – actions.

Pressor action of Adr is reversed by = **phentolamine;** which is an alpha-blocker. It is ka **vasomotor reversal of Dale**. Alpha receptors mainly lie in pre and post- junctional neurons which are blocked by phentolamine. Decreased PR → decreased CO → decreased B P due to beta-mediated vasodilation.

Mechanism of action = alpha receptors operate by modifying ionic permeability. Beta receptors operate by increasing cAMP levels.

Parasympathetic

1. Cholinergic = Ach; muscarine; pilocarpine etc.
2. Anticholinesterase = physiostigmine; neostigmine; organophosphate etc.
3. Anticholinergic = atropine; hyoscine/scopolamine; propantheline; tricyclic antidepressants; phenothiazine derivatives; antihistaminics etc.
4. Adrenergic = ka catecholamines; e.g. adr, n- adr; dopamine; ephedrine; isoprenaline etc.; phenylephrine.
5. Alpha – blockers = phenoxybenzamine; ergotamine; ergotoxin; chlorpromazine; phentolamine; prazosine etc.;
6. Beta – blockers = propranolol; atenolol; labetolol etc.

Alpha stimulation = vasoconstriction
Beta stimulation = vasodilation
Beta 1 = cardiac stimulation
Beta 2 = bronchodilation

Cholinergic receptors

Nicotinic = on skeletal muscles—contract; autonomic ganglia – stimulate.

Muscarinic = on neuroeffector junctions of para-SNS. Eg heart (decrease HR, force); blood vessels (decrease BP, dilate); eye (miosis).

Sympathetic ganglia = have both nicotinic and cholinergic receptors.

GENERAL ANAESTHESIA

- GA used in hemorrhagic shock = cycloprocaine
- For **bloodless field** = **halothane,** causes CVS depression and hepatic necrosis.
- **Sense depressed last** by GA = hearing
- Enflurane is indicated when Adr is given for bloodless field.
- **Last vital function to be depressed** by GA = CVS function, which is a sequlae of respiratory paralysis.
- Fluothane = best GA for an **asthmatic** patient, a **bronchodilator**
- Norepinephrine = most effective in activating alpha – receptors
- Beta adrenergic receptors are closely related to = adenylate cyclase enzyme, which increases cAMP.
- Muscarinic receptors are associated with = guanyl cyclase, which increases cGMP.
- Halothane = causes **liver damage**
- Cyclopropane = sensitizes patient's **myocardium** to catecholamines
- N_2O above 80% can lead to hypoxia.
- **Malignant hyperthermia** is caused by enzyme deficiency in a patient on GA by persistent release of Ca ++ from sarcoplasmic reticulum. It is treated by **dentrolene sodium.**
- **Neuroadaptation** = i.e. physical dependence of a drug
- **Dissociated analgesia** = ketamine iv, ethylate iv
- Ketamine = produces profound analgesia without disturbing respiratory and CVS functions, produces **dissociative anaesthesia**, used in **children**

- **Neurolept anaesthesia** = combination of antipsychotic drug with schedule II drug e.g. fentanyl – droperidol combination. Droperidol is antipsychotic. C/I in impaired respiration.
- **Lytic cocktail** = promethazine + chlorpromazine + meperidine; is for conscious sedation. (PCM)
- N_2O causes = **methemoglobulinemia**
- Depth of GA depends on the potency of the agent.
- **Vital centers** located in medulla are paralysed the last with the increasing depth of anaesthesia.
- Conc of GA agent is more in white matter than in grey matter.

STAGES OF GA

Stage I = stage of analgesia = only short procedure can be done; pain is gradually abolished during this stage.

Stage II = stage of delirium = excitement is seen; pupils dilate; **no stimulus is applied or any** surgery is done in it.

Stage III = surgical anaesthesia = divided in 4 planes = most of the **surgical procedures are done** ; esp within planes 1 and 2.

- **Plane 1** = roving eyeballs; ends when eyes become fixed; pupils normal size;
- **Plane 2** = loss of corneal and laryngeal reflexes; pupils normal size
- **Plane 3** = pupil starts dilating and light reflex is lost
- **Plane 4** = dilated pupils; intercostal paralysis

Stage IV = medullary paralysis = respiration stops; death; pupils widely dilated; BP very low; skeletal ms are flabby as tone is lost.

Summary

Stage I	Pupils normal; respiration normal; BP/ HR normal;	Minor surgery; labour
Stage II; excitement	Pupils dilate; involuntary skeletal ms movements;	No surgery

Summary (*Contd.*)

Planes 1, 2	Normal pupils; corneal and laryngeal reflexes lost	Most of the surgical procedures are done
Plane 3	Light reflex is lost; pupils dilate	
Plane 4 Stage IV	Dilated pupils; Widely dilated pupils; loss of skeletal ms tone; BP/ HR nil	Death due to respiratory failure

Inhalation sedation

- Most common agent used is N_2O with O_2 gas.
- Commonest delivery system used is Quantiflex system.

  Guedel classification of anesthesia describes 3 stages
  - Stage 1 = analgesia
  - Stage 2 = excitement
  - Stage 3 = surgical anesthesia
- First stage of anesthesia can be divided into 3 planes

  Plane 1 = moderate sedation, some analgesia; 15 – 35 % N_2O.

  Plane 2 = dissociation: increasing analgesia, 25 – 55 % N_2O

  Plane 3 = total analgesia prior to loss of conciousness; > 55% N_2O.
- 15 – 30 % N_2O plane 1 inhalational sedation
- 25 – 35 % N_2O plane 2 relative analgesia
- > 55 % N_2O plane 3 total analgesia; unconsciousness.

NITROUS OXIDE

1. Discovered by Priestlay in 1776.
2. It is stored in a BLUE cylinder.

3. It is always used in combination of O_2 gas. 70 % N_2O + 25 – 30 % O_2 gas is generally used. It helps in better m/m of respiration and circulation functions rather than the GA agent given alone.
4. Onset action is quick and smooth.
5. Widely used in **pediatric dentistry.**

ETHER

1. It causes **marked ms relaxation** by reducing acetylcholine output form the motor nerve endings.
2. Atropine must be given as premedication to prevent secretions.

   Premedication = laryngospasm can be prevented by atropine premedication; as the secretions are decreased.

HALOTHANE

1. It is not a good analgesic or ms relaxant agent.
2. It causes direct depression of myocardial contractility by reducing intracellular Ca^{++} concentration.
3. It is **preferred for asthmatics** because it causes early abolition of pharyngeal and laryngeal reflexes and dilates the bronchi.
4. S/E = may cause **malignant hyperthermia**; its Rx of choice is **dentrolene sodium** i.v.
5. Succinylcholine increases the malignant hyperthermia caused by halothane.
6. It may cause serious cardiac irregularities in p.o epinephrine, as it sensitizes heart to arrythmogenic action of Adr.

ISOFLURANE = has **least effect on CVS;** it is preferred for **neurosurgery** as it does not provoke seizures.

THIOPENTONE SODIUM = it is the last drug to be used in cases of status epilepticus patients; the anaesthetic action of benzodiazepines can be rapidly **reversed by flumazenil**.

It should be freshly prepared before injection.

KETAMINE = it induces dissociative anaesthesia, **used in children** mainly; effect lasts for 10 – 15 min.; esp useful for **burn dressings**; causes sympathetic stimulations. Its **primary site of action** is cortex and subcortical areas. It does not cause unconsciousness.

FENTANYL – DROPERIDOL COMBINATION

It causes **neurolept analgesia**; it can be changed to neurolept anaesthesia by administering 65 % N_2O + 35 % O_2 gas.

Analeptics = are the drugs which stimulate respiration and can **have resuscitative values in coma or fainting**.

Pre-anaesthetic medications

- Opioids = morphine or pethidine i.m., allay anxiety and apprehension, makes patient calm, smoothens the induction
- Promethazine = antihistaminic properties; used esp in children as it has little respiratory depression.
- Glycopyrrolate = antisecretory and antibradycardiac actions;
- Metoclopramide = enhances gastric emptying and tone of lower esophageal sphincter; reduces chances of reflux.

ANTIBIOTICS

1. **Sulfonamides** = mechanism of action is by inhibition of **bacterial folate synthetase enzyme**.

   Metabolised in liver, excreted by kidney.

   Special drugs = sulfasalazine = used in **ulcerative colitis** and rheumatoid arthritis;

   Mafenide = used topically mainly **in burns dressing** to prevent infection

   Sulfacetamide sodium = used topically for ocular infections.

   S/E = hypersensitivity; **Stevens – Jhonson syndrome** occurs usually with long acting sulfonamides. **Hemolysis** in patients having G6PD deficiency.

   Cotrimoxazole is the drug of choice for uncomplicated UTI except enterococcus.

2. **Trimethoprim** = acts by inhibiting **bacterial dihydrofolate reductase** enz.

   When used with sulfamethoxazole, it causes sequential block of folate metabolism.

Ratio of sulfamethoxazole and trimethoprim **is 5 : 1.**

It may cause **folate deficiency anemia.**

3. **Penicillins** = mech of action = they interfere with the synthesis of **bacterial cell wall** by inhibiting transpeptidases and carboxypeptidases s.t. cross linking of nucleotides does not occur. G (+) bacteria having **peptidoglycan cell wall** are very sensitive to it; are hydrolysed by beta – lactamase enz and so are ineffective vs the organisms producing the **beta – lactamase**.

   Penicillin – G is narrow spectrum antibiotic, active vs G (+) bacteria;

   It is the **drug of choice** in syphilis, group A and B Strept infections, actinomycosis, oral and PDL infections, strept. viridans endocarditis; tetanus, etc.

   Penicillinase resistant penicillins e.g. **methicullin** are drug of choice for **staphylococcal infections.**

   The resistance is acquired through the production of penicillinase.

   When **beta – lactamase inhibitors** e.g. clavulanic acid or sulbactam are added to ampicillin, amoxicillin, etc. the spectrum is improved.

   Penicillin given to the secondary syphilitic patient may cause Jarisch Herxheimer reaction.

CEPHALOSPORINS

Second generation cephalosporins are not active against pseudomonas or acinectobactor.

3rd generation drugs are broad spectrum and are active vs gram negative rods; esp useful **in hospital acquired infections**. But they have no activity vs methicillin resistant – staph, etc.

Tetracycline

- broad spectrum, **bacteriostatic agents**
- active vs G + and G – bacteria.
- Highest incidence of **photosensitivity** is seen with **demeclocycline** and doxycycline.
- Calcium – tetracycline chelates may get deposited in teeth and bone causing brown discoloration during the mineralization state.

- Tetracycline if given b/w 3 mos to 5 yrs age children affects the permanent teeth.
- Demeclocycline may **cause diabetes insipidus**.
- **Except doxycycline,** all tetracyclines are **excreted in urine** by glomerular filtration.
- **Doxycycline** is mainly metabolized and **excreted in feces as** conjugate.
- **Minocycline** is mainly metabolized and excreted **in urine and bile**.
- Are the most common antibiotics **causing superinfections,** as they cause marked suppression of the resident flora.
- It should not be used in pregnancy, lactation and children below 8 yrs age.

Chloramphenicol

- Is a bacteriostatic agent; produced from **actinomycetes**.
- Resistance vs it is due to plasmid encoded enz, i.e. chloramphenicol acetyl transferase
- Causes irreversible **bone marrow depression;**
- Ciprofloxacin is the drug of choice for typhoid fever now. **Ceftriaxone** is the fastest acting drug vs typhoid fever. Also ceftriaxone is the **best choice in children**.
- In neonates, it causes **gray baby syndrome;** may occur in high doses.

Aminoglycosides

- Streptomycin was the first aminoglycoside; is obtained from **streptomyces griseus.**
- Are produced **by soil actinomycetes;** excreted unchanged in urine;
- **Ototoxicity** = conc. dependent destructive changes occur; destroy the hair cells within inner ear causing permanent damage.
- **Nephrotoxicity** = due to peritubular accumulation of aminoglycosides and causes proximal tubular damage. **Streptomycin has least nephrotoxicity.**
- They cause nm blockade by **reducing acetylcholine release** from motor nerve endings. And so prolongs the action of curare like

muscle relaxants. Tobromycin causes least nm blockade. It can be partially antagonized by **i.v calcium**.

- They are combined with beta – lactam antibiotics for Rx of G (-) septicemia.

Macrolides

- Erythromycin is broad spectrum vs G + bacteria.
- GIT S/E are due to binding of the drug with **motilin** receptors causing **increased gut motility.**

Quinolones

- Are synthetic antimicrobials.
- **Nalidixic acid is the** first member of the group; acts by inhibiting bacterial DNA replication.
- Most imp side effects s/e are **neurological.**
- Fluoroquinolones = mech. of action is by inhibition of DNA – gyrase; ciprofloxacin has widest spectrum and is most potent; ciprofloxacin is the **most active vs pseudomonas.**
- Nofloxacin is used vs UTI; genital tract infections and infectious diarrhoea.

Metronidazole

- Active vs anaerobic and protozoa organisms.
- It is the **drug of choice for any abscess** where obligate anaerobic infection is suspected.
- It is the drug of choice for amoebiasis etc.
- It should not be used in **first 3 months of pregnancy** due to its suspected mutagenic and teratogenic effects.
- It acts by **inhibiting DNA synthesis.**
- It inhibits the cell mediated immunity/CMI.

ANTIVIRAL DRUGS

Interferons

- Prepared by DNA recombinant technology.
- Interferon **alpha 2 b is** used in Rx of chronic hepatitis B, non A and non B.

- Hairy cell leukemia, Kaposi's sarcoma is treated by interferon alpha 2 a and alpha 2 b.

Acyclovir

- MOA = by inhibiting virus induced DNA polymerase. Also gets incorporated in viral DNA causing **early chain termination.**
- Mostly used in Rx of **genital H. simplex** infection.
- When used in AIDS repeatedly, it may lead to resistant strains of H. simplex and VZV, which can respond to **Foscarnet**. Mech of action of foscarnet is that it acts by inhibiting viral DNA polymerase at the pyrophosphate binding sites.
- **Zidovudine** = inhibits the replication of HIV thro the competitive **inhibition of HIV reverse transcriptase** and thro the chain termination of viral DNA synthesis.
- **Vidarbine** = acts by inhibition of viral DNA synthesis.

Important points

Aluminium hydroxide causes constipation whereas magnesium hydroxide causes loose stools.

Hydrogen blockers = used to inhibit the gastric acid / HCl secretion. And used for Rx of **peptic ulcers**.

ADH/vasopressin = is synthesised by nerve cell bodies in hypothalamus.

Desmopressin is a selective V_2 receptor antagonist and is the drug of choice in **diabetes insipidus.**

Hb contains about 3 mg of iron which is recycled 10 times daily.

Inorganic iron is mostly in ferric form. It needs to be **reduced to ferrous form before absorption**.

Specific antidote for *iron poisoning* is = desferrioxamine.

Most common side effect of oral iron therapy is = constipation.

Anticoagulants

Heparin is the strongest organic acid present in the body.

Heparin is present in all tissues containing mast cells.

Heparin acts by activating plasma antithrombin III, blocks the action of factor X and thrombin.

Specific **antidote of heparin** = protamine sulphate

Oral anticoagulants

They are **competitive antagonist of vit K.**

Act by interfering with the regeneration of active hydroquinone form of vit K.

Specific antidote of oral anticoagulant is = vit K 1.

Dose of oral anticoagulant is regulated by = PT

It is **C/I in pregnancy** due to risk of **birth defects developments**.

Warfarin = acts by inhibiting the synthesis of clotting factors.

Fibrinolysis = is an imp part of the normal hemostatic process; it is initiated by the release of either TPA, i.e. tissue plasminogen activator or pro-urokinase from the endothelial cells.

Tranexaemic acid and EACA are **anti-fibrinolytic drugs.** They inhibit plasminogen activators and dissolution of clots.

Antiplatelet therapy = **aspirin** is the most common drug used for it. It causes inactivation of enz cycloxygenase and so inhibition of production of thromboxane - A 2 by platelets.

AUTONOMIC NERVOUS SYSTEM

- all organs have ANS **except skeletal ms.**
- Preganglionic nerve fibres **are myelinated**; postganglionic fibres are non – myelinated; somatic fibres are myelinated.
- Anterior and medial nuclei of hypothalamus control parasympathetic, but posterior and lateral nuclei are sympathetic.
- Most blood vessels, spleen, sweat glands, and hair follicles = receive **only sympathetic** innervation.
- Ciliary ms, gastric and pancreatic glands receive = **only parasympathetic innervation**.
- *Acetylcholine* is the major neurotransmitter at autonomic and somatic sites.
- *Acetylcholinesterase* is present in all cholinergic sites, RBCs, grey matter and is inhibited by physostigmine.

- All blood vessels have muscarinic receptors located on endothelial cells, they cause smooth ms relaxation.
- Hyoscine or *scopolamine* is the most effective **drug for motion sickness**.
- Rx of *atropine poisoning* is gastric lavage done with **tannic acid**.
- Insulin dependent diabetes mellitus (IDDM) = probably is an **autoimmune** disease; more prone to **ketosis**; hereditary also.
- Diabetic ketoacidosis or diabetic coma occurs in IDDM generally and the **main cause is infection.**
- NIDDM = there is **no loss of beta – cells;** circulating insulin is normal / high.
- **Somatostatin** inhibits release of insulin and glucagon.
- Insulin inhibits glucagon secretion. (Insulin has action opposite of glucagon).
- Insulin facilitates glucose transport across the cell membrane.
- **Benzodiazepines** = act preferentially on midbrain ascending **reticular formation**, which maintains wakefulness, and **on limbic system** /, i.e. thought and mental functions. They have only GABA facilitatory function. Antidote is **flumazenil.**
- **Aspirin** = inhibits prostaglandin synthesis and blocks the sensitization of pain mechanism. Antipyretic action of aspirin is related to **inhibition of PG synthesis**. It reduces fever by promoting heat loss/ sweating. It is ulcerogenic as it causes back diffusion of acid in mucosa. It is recommended in heart disease.
- **Allopurinol** = is the **uric acid synthesis inhibitor;** it is a competitive inhibitor of **xanthine oxidase**. R_x of gout.
- **Cocaine** = should never be injected; only **surface anaesthesia;** used only in **ocular anaesthesia**; is sympathomimetic it increases BP and HR; powerful CNS stimulant; psychostimulant; vasoconstrictor.
- CNS depressants decrease the levels of mediators in ganglia. Eg Chlorpromazine decreases dopamine levels; diazepam decreases GABA levels.
- CNS stimulants = increases the level of mediators e.g. amphetamine.

- Sympathetic supply to heart is stimulatory; **vagus is inhibitory** to heart.
- H_1 blockers = anti-histaminics; act by **competitive antagonism** with histamine at H_1 – receptors.
- H_2 blockers = e.g. cimetidine competitively inhibits histamine induced gastric secretions.
- Use of vasoconstrictor in combination with LA is C/I in a dental patient who is = with **parkinsonism disease** and is on levodopa therapy as shown below that levels of N.Adr increase then.
- Levodopa → dopamine → N Adr.
- Parkinsonism is due to **deficiency of dopamine** / DA; DA is depleted by reserpine;
- D – tubocurarine = is a peripherally acting ms relaxant.
- Propranolol is C/I in = cardiac arrythmias.
- Thiazides increase the toxicity of digitalis. Digitalis causes decreased conc of K^+ ions in heart ms; thiazides cause renal excretion of K^+ so they cause decreased levels of K^+ in blood.
- **Chlorthiazide act** on cortical diluting segment **of loop of Henle** or early distal tubules. They inhibit Na+ reabsorption; Cl^- and water are retained in the tubule secondarily. Also, decreased GFR, renal Ca^{++} excretion, urate excretion and increased Mg^{++} excretion and increased blood sugar due to decreased insulin release occurs. So, hyponatremia; hypokalemia; hyperuricemia; hypercalcemia and hyperglycemia occurs.

GENERAL PHARMACOLOGY

- Pharmacodynamics = i.e. what the drug does to the body.
- Pharmacokinetics = i.e. what the body does to the drug.
- Clinical pharmacology = is the scientific study of drugs in man. Its aim is to generate data for optimum use of drugs.
- Pharmacodynamic agent = are assigned to have pharmacodynamic effects in the recipient.
- Chemotherapeutic agents = are designed to kill / inhibit invading parasites / malignant cells.

Routes of drug administration

- Oral = commonest route; non – invasive; slow action.
- **Sublingual** = **only lipid – soluble drugs** can be given; **liver is byepassed** and so drugs with high first pass metabolism are absorbed directly in systemic circulation. Action is relatively **rapid**. Eg nitroglycerine; nifedipine etc.
- Cutaneous = **highly lipid soluble** drugs can be applied for slow and prolonged absorption. Liver is bye passed.
- Inhalation = action is **very rapid;** controlled; e.g. GA agents, amylnitrite etc.
- Parenteral = drug deposited directly in the blood or tissue fluid; **faster and surer action**; **liver is bye passed;** controlled;
- I/V = great value in **emergencies;** only **aqueous solutions** should be injected; dose required is smallest; 100 % bioavailability;
- I/M = ms are more vascular; so absorption is faster; less painful;
- Intradermal = i.e. in skin raising a bleb; e.g. BCG, small pox vaccines; for sensitivity testing;

PHARMACOKINETICS

- Is the **qualitative study of drug movement** in, through, and out of the body.
- It involves transport of the drug across the biological membranes (which is a bilayer of lipid molecules).
- **Passive diffusion** = i.e. drug diffuses in the direction of its concentration gradient.
- A **more lipid soluble drug attains higher concentration** in membrane and diffuses quickly.
- A pH difference across a membrane can cause differential distribution of weakly acidic and basic drugs on the 2 sides.
- Basic drugs attain higher concentration intracellularly (pH 7.0 vs 7.4 of plasma)
- Acidic drugs are unionised at acidic pH of stomach and get **absorbed there**, while basic drugs largely ionised and are absorbed only when they reach the intestine., i.e. absorption of ionised drugs does not occur.

- Acidic drugs get more ionised in alkaline urine and get excreted faster.
- Basic drugs excreted faster in acidified urine .

Active transport – occurs vs the concentration gradient.

Facilitated transport – it translocates nondiffusible substrates along their conc gradient and *does not need energy.* It is more rapid.

Pinocytosis = i.e. transport across the cell in **the particulate form** by formation of vesicles.

Absorption of drugs – if taken orally -

- The epithelial *lining of GIT is* **lipoidal** so the non – ionised lipid soluble drugs are readily absorbed.
- Faster gastric emptying accelerates drug absorption.
- Tetracyclines form complexes with Ca++ and absorption gets delayed chelation occur.
- Lipid insoluble drugs do not enter cells.
- Drugs extensively bound to plasma proteins are largely restricted to the **vascular compartment** and have low values of distribution.

Redistribution

- **Highly lipid soluble drugs** given i/v, inhalation first go to organs with high blood flow and then get redistributed to less vascular but more bulky tissues e.g. ms, fat.
- Thiopentone action gets terminated in a few minutes due to redistribution.

Blood brain barrier = i.e. capillary endothelial linings have tight junctions and is lined by a sheet of **glial cells**.

Blood – CSF barrier = is located in **choroid plexus.**

BBB and BCB are **lipoidal** and limit entry of non-lipid soluble drugs.

So only **lipid soluble drugs can penetrate and have action on CNS** e.g. levodopa enters brain and used for Rx of parkinsonism.

At CTZ in medulla, = the barrier is deficient and so even lipid insoluble drugs are emetic.

The action of **ultra – short acting barbiturates is** terminated primarily by the process of = *redistribution;* they have **high lipid solubility**; fat is saturated in the last.

Placental barrier = **placenta is lipoidal** and so lipid soluble/ lipophilic drugs cross it. It is an **incomplete barrier**. Fluoride can cross it practically.

Plasma – protein binding

1. Acidic drugs bind to albumin.
2. Basic drugs bind to alpha – 1 acid glycoproteins.
3. Highly plasma protein bound drugs **get largely restricted to vascular compartment** and has lower volumes of distribution and **become longer acting.**
4. Bound fraction is not available for action.

Tissues storage

Drugs may accumulate in specific organs e.g.

- Skeletal ms / heart — emetine
- Thyroid — iodine
- Retina — chloroquine
- Iris — atropine (bound to melanin)
- Bones / teeth — tetracycline / heavy metals

To specific tissue constituents

- Tetracycline — to mitochondria
- Chloroquine — to nuclei

BIOTRANSFORMATION = metabolism is required to **make lipid soluble compounds the non-lipid soluble** so that they are not reabsorbed in renal tubules and are excreted. Primary site of drug metabolism is LIVER.

Prodrug = i.e. few drugs are inactive as such and need conversion in the body to active metabolite.

First pass / presystemic metabolism = i.e. metabolism of drug during its passage from intestines to the systemic circulation.

Basic drugs are more **conc in breast milk**.

Urine is the most imp channel of excretion for most drugs.

Lipid soluble drugs get **reabsorbed in the renal tubules**, but non-lipid soluble and highly ionised drugs are unable to do so and get excreted.

Weak bases ionise more and is less reabsorbed in acidic urine.

Weak acids ionise more and is less reabsorbed in alkaline urine.

KINETICS OF ELIMINATION

1. **First order / exponential kinetics** = i.e. rate of elimination is directly proportional to the drug conc, i.e. ***a constant fraction of the drug*** present in the body is eliminated in unit time, i.e. **clearance remains constant.**
2. **Zero order / linear kinetics** = rate of elimination remains constant irrespective of the drug conc, **clearance decreases** with the increase in conc, i.e. ***a constant amount of drug is eliminated*** in unit time e.g. ethyl alcohol.
3. **Clearance** = is the volume of plasma from which the drug is completely removed in a unit time., e.g. creatinine clearance.
4. **Plasma half life** = i.e. the time taken for its plasma conc. to be reduced to half of its original value. $T\ \frac{1}{2} = 0.693 \times \text{volume} / \text{clearance}$. **Nearly complete drug elimination occurs in 4 – 5 half lives.**

For drugs eliminated by first order kinetics = t ½ is constant as V and Clearance does not change.

For drugs eliminated by zero order kinetics = t ½ increases with dose as clearance progressively decreases.

PHARMACODYNAMICS

1. **INHIBITION** = Of enzymes is a common method of drug action.
2. **Competitive inhibition** = i.e. drug competes with normal substrate or coenzymes s.t. a new equilibrium is achieved in p.o drug.

3. **Non –competitive** = i.e. inhibitor reacts with adjacent site and not with catalytic site and alters the enzyme s.t it loses its catalytic property.
4. **Agonist** = it **activates a receptor** to produce an effect. It has both affinity and maximal intrinsic activity.
5. **Antagonist** = prevents action of an agonist on a receptor or the subsequent response but has no effect of its own.
6. **Partial agonist** = activates a receptor to produce submaximal effect but antagonises the action of a full agonist.

Affinity = is the **ability of** the drug to combine with the receptors.

Efficacy = maximum **response** elicited by a drug

Potency = **amount of** drug required to produce a certain response

Therapeutic index = LD 50 / ED 50

7. **Intrinsic activity / efficacy** = is the ability to activate / induce a confirmational change in the receptor.
8. **Agonist** = It has both affinity and maximal intrinsic activity.
9. **Competitive antagonist** = have affinity but no intrinsic activity.
10. **Partial agonist** = have affinity and submaximal intrinsic activity.

	Affinity	Intrinsic activity
Agonist	Yes	Maximal
Competitive agonist	Yes	No
Partial agonist	Yes	Submaximal

Drug action = is the initial combination of the drug with its receptor resulting in a confirmational change in the receptor.

Drug effect = is the ultimate change in biological function due to drug action thro a series of intermediate steps.

Drug potency = is the amount of drug required to produce a certain response.

Efficacy of drug is the **maximal response** that can be elicited by the drug.

Efficacy is a more decisive factor in the choice of a drug.

Therapeutic index / safety margin = TI = median lethal dose / median effective dose, i.e. LD 50 / ED 50.

Combined effects of the drugs

1. **Synergism** = action of one drug is facilitated or increased by the other.
2. **Additive** = effects of 2 drugs simply add up, i.e. action of (A +B) = action of A + action of B.
3. **Supra additive / potentiation** = effect of combination is more than the individual effects of the components, i.e. (A + B) > (A) + (B).
4. **Antagonism** = i.e. one drug decreases or inhibits the action of other, i.e. (A + B) < (A) + (B).

- 2 drugs may have opposite effects on same physiological function or their pharmacological actions are in opposite directions.
- **Receptor antagonism** = i.e. antagonist interferes with binding of agonist with its receptor; it is **specific.**
- **Physiological / functional antagonism** = 2 drugs have pharmacological **effects in opposite directions**, e.g. histamine and Adr on BP / bronchial ms.
- **Competitive antagonism** = i.e. antagonist binds with **the same receptor as** the agonist and the antagonist chemically resembles the agonist. Antagonist reduces affinity/potency of agonist, e.g. Ach – atropine combination.
- **Chemical antagonism** = 2 drugs **react chemically** and form an inactive product.
- **Non – competitive** = antagonist binds **with another receptor** site and reduces the efficacy/intrinsic activity of agonist; it does not resemble agonist chemically.

DRUG DOSAGES

Dose of drug is governed by its inherent potency, i.e. its conc at target site.

Standard dose = has a wide safety margin; same dose is appropriate for most patients.

Regulated dose = dose is accurately adjusted by repeated measurement of the affected physiological parameters.

DOSAGE CALCULATION

- **Clark's rule** = child dose = $\frac{\text{child weight (lbs)}}{150} \times$ adult dose
- % of A.D = 0.7 × wt. of the child
- Child dose = wt (kgs) × AD / 70
- Child dose = surface area (m^2) × AD / 1.7
- **Young's rule** = CD = age × AD / (age + 12)
- **Dilling's rule** = CD = age × AD / 20

In elderly, the renal function progressively declines and drug doses have to be decreased.

Blood brain barrier is more **permeable in newborns**.

Hepatic drug metabolising system is inadequate in newborns, e.g. chloramphenicol can produce **gray – baby syndrome**.

Permeability of blood brain barrier is **increased in renal failure**.

Certain drugs worsen existing clinical conditions in renal failure, e.g. tetracyclines **except doxycycline,** have anti-anabolic effect and so increases uremia.

HYPOTHYROID PATIENTS are **more sensitive to digoxin,** morphine and other CNS depressants.

Hyperthyroids are relatively **resistant to** inotropic action but more prone to arrhythmic action of digoxin.

MI patients are more prone to Adr and digitalis induced cardiac arrythmia.

Myasthenics are very sensitive to curare.

Morphine should be avoided in head – injury otherwise respiratory failure.

Diabetics receiving insulin / sulfonyl ureas may develop asymptomatic but **dangerous hypoglycemia** if propranolol is added.

Aspirin decreases K + conserving action of spironolactone.

Tolerance = is requirement of **higher doses** of a drug to produce a given response.

Cross tolerance = is development of tolerance to a pharmacologically related drug.

Tachyphylaxis = is the **rapid development of tolerance**. Its usually seen with indirectly acting drugs.

Drug resistance = is the tolerance of microbes to inhibiting action of antibiotics.

UNIVERSAL ANTIDOTE = burned toast + strong tea + milk in 2:1:1 ratio.

Idiosyncracy = is genetically determined **abnormal reactivity** to a chemical.

Drug allergy = is immunologically mediated reaction producing stereotyped symptoms which are **unrelated to pharmacodynamics** of the drug and is largely independent of the dose. It is aka **hypersensitivity.**

Supersensitivity = is an **increased response** to a drug.

Hapten/incomplete Ag = i.e. small molecules which become antigenic only after binding with endogenous protein.

Reactions are:

1. **Humoral / Ab –mediated**
   - Type I / anaphylactic reaction
   - Type II / cytolytic
   - Type III / retarded / Arthus reactions
2. **Cell mediated** =
   - Type IV / delayed hypersensitivity

Type I = reaginic Abs (IgE) + mast cells → + Ag → histamines, 5-HT, PGs, SRS-A; so quick reactions occur ka **immediate hypersensitivity**.

Type II = (IgG, IgM + target cells) → + re-exposure to Ag → C' is activated → **cytolysis**, e.g. thrombocytopenia, agranulocytosis, hemolysis etc.

Type III = by IgG and circulating Abs **(mopping Abs)**

Ag – Ab complex + C' → precipitates **on endothelial linings** of blood vessels → inflammation ; e.g. serum sickness, polyarteritis nodosa, LAP, erythema multiforme, arthralgia, myocarditis etc.

This reaction usually subsides in 1 – 2 wks.

Type IV = occurs through T – cells.

Ag + T – cells → lymphokines are released → attract **granulocytes** → response is generated; eg contact dermatitis, photosensitisation etc.

Phototoxic = drugs/metabolites get accumulated in skin and absorb light; lead to **local tissue damage;** esp shorter wavelengths (290 - 320 nm), e.g. tetracyclines esp **demeclocycline** and tar – products.

Photoallergic = by 320- 400 nm, UV-A; cell mediated response; contact dermatitis – like picture.

Physical dependence = aka **neuroadaptation**

- Continued p.o. drug is required to maintain physiological equilibrium.
- Discontinuation leads to withdrawl/**abstinence syndrome.**
- Produced mainly by CNS – depressants; (very little by CNS stimulant drugs, e.g. amphetamine, cocaine; these produce drug – addiction.)

Teratogenicity = i.e. drugs causing **fetal abnormalities;** most vulnerable period is stage of organogenesis; 18 – 55 days i.u., e.g.

- Thalidomide = phocomelia
- Corticosteroids = CLP
- Tetracyclines = discolor the teeth/ retarded bone growth/
- Aspirin = premature closure of **ductus arteriosus**
- Indomethacin = premature closure of **ductus arteriosus**

Differences b/w sympathetic nervous system and para- sympathetic nervous system:

Property	SNS	PNS
Origin	T1 – L2,3, i.e. thoraco lumbar	Craniosacral = 3,7,9, 10 + S, 2-4
Ganglia Post-gang fibres	Away from the organs Long	Close to the organ Short
Pre : Post gang fibre ratio	1: 20 to 1: 100	1:1to 1: 2
Transmitters	Major = N-Adr Minor = Ach	**Ach only;** gets locally degraded
Functions	Tackling stress and emergency	Assimilation of food and conservation of energy

Somatic nervous system

- Supplies skeletal ms
- Fibres are myelinated
- Ach is the transmitter substance
- No peripheral plexus is formed

ANS

- Supplies all the other organs **except skeletal** ms.
- Pre ganglionic fibres are myelinated; post ganglionic fibres are non – myelinated.
- Ach and N Adr are the transmitters.
- Peripheral plexus is formed.

Autonomic efferents = cell bodies lie **in dorsal root ganglia** of spinal nerves and sensory ganglia of cranial ns; they mediate visceral pain and reflexes.

Central autonomic connections = mainly hypothalamus.

- Posterior and lateral nuclei = sympathetic
- Anterior and medial nuclei = para sympathetic
- Lateral column in thoracic spinal cord = sympathetic outflow.

Autonomic efferents = 2 subdivisions = sympathetic and p – sympathetic; which are **functionally antagonistic.**

Most blood vessels / spleen / sweat glands/ hair follicles receive only = sympathetic supply.

Ciliary ms/ gastric and pancreatic glands = receive only para-sympathetic supply.

Resting transmembrane potential = - 70 mV inside by active Na^+ extrusion.

During reverse polarisation = inside becomes + 20 mV;

In refractory period = activation of Na – K pump occurs.

Tetrodotoxin and saxitoxin = selectively abolish Na+ conductance in nerve fibres and block the impulse conduction.

ACETYL CHOLINE

- Major neurotransmitter at both, i.e. somatic and autonomic sites.
- Synthesised from **choline** and acetyl CoA in p.o. enz choline acetylase.
- **Hemicholinium blocks choline** uptake and depletes Ach.
- It is immediately **destroyed locally by enz cholinesterase;** its reuptake does not occur.
- 2 toxins interfere with cholinergic transmission are

  botulinum toxin = inhibits release

  black widow spider toxin = induces massive release and depletion.

16

MCQs in Pharmacology

1. **All of the following are currently accepted as neurotransmitters in the CNS *except***
   A. Acetylcholine
   B. Dopamine
   C. Nor epinephrine
   D. Reserpine
   E. Serotonin
   F. GABA (gamma-aminobutyric acid)
   G. Opioid peptides (beta endorphin enkephalins and dynorphin)
   H. Glycine
   I. Glutamate and aspartate

2. **What are the four criteria to consider when selecting an analgesic agent for a patient?**
   A. Type of pain
   B. Location of pain
   C. Age of patient
   D. Sex of patient
   E. Patient's mental state
   F. Concurrent medication
   G. Pregnancy

3. **An IV injection of histamine results in all of the following except.**
   A. A fall in systemic blood pressure
   B. An increase in gastric acid secretion
   C. Constriction of CNS blood vessels
   D. Bronchoconstriction
   E. Dilation of terminal arterioles

4. All of the following statements concerning rennin are true *except.*

A. Renin is an enzyme that is produced by and stored in the granular cells of the juxtaglomerular apparatus of the kidneys.
B. It is released by granular cells of the kidney into the blood in response to sodium depletion and/or low blood volume
C. Renin converts angiotensin I to angiotensin II
D. High levels of renin in the blood may indicate Addison's disease, cirrhosis, essential hypertension, hypokalemia, malignant hypertension of Barter's syndrome

5. The prototype tricyclic antidepressant drug is

A. Imipramine
B. Amitriptyline
C. Desipramine
D. Nortriptyline
E. Clomipramine
F. Doxepin
G. Protriptyline

6. Chloramphenicol is active against all of the following except

A. Gram-positive bacteria
B. Gram-negative bacteria
C. Anaerobic bacteria
D. Fungi
E. Rickettsia

7. Which of the following is a contraindication or precaution to the use of prilocaine ?

A. Biliary tract disease
B. Imipenem hypersensitivity
C. Benzyl alcohol hypersensitivity
D. Hepatic disease

8. All of the following anti epileptic drugs are effective in treating absence seizures (formerly called petitmal) except.

A. Ethosuximide
B. Valproic acid
C. Phenytoin
D. Clonazepam

9. **All of the following are important effects of aspirin (acetylsalicylic acid) except**
   A. The reduction of fever
   B. The reduction of prostaglandin synthesis in inflamed tissue
   C. The reduction of the tendency to bleed
   D. Respiratory stimulation when taken in toxic dosage
   E. Tinnitus and vertigo

10. **All of the following are anti-muscarinic agents except**
   A. Atropine
   B. Scopolamine
   C. Glycopyrrolate
   D. Mecamylamine
   E. Methantheline
   F Propantheline

11. **Poisoning with an organophosphate cholinesterase inhibitor can be treated with**
   A. Edrophonium
   B. Carbachol
   C. Pralidoxime
   D. Nicotine

12. **Which of the following can develop during therapy with phenobarbital**
   A. Drowsiness
   B. Dizziness
   C. Lethargy
   D. Headache
   E. Vertigo
   F. Severe depression
   G. Anxiety
   H. Irritability
   I. All of the above

13. **The drug of choice in anaphylaxis is**
   A. Nor epinephrine
   B. Terbutaline
   C. Epinephrine
   D. Phenycephrine

14. Of the following, which is a clinically significant adverse reaction due to Metoprolol?

A. Alopecia
B. Dry mouth
C. Dysarthria
D. Folliculits

15. The most common adverse effect associated with the benzodiazepines include all of the following except

A. Ataxia
B. CNS depression (drowsiness and sedation)
C. Confusion
D. Disorientation
E. Dry mouth
F. GI disturbances (nausea, vomiting and diarrhoea)

16. Which of the drugs are considered to be anti arrhythmic agents?

A. Sodium channel blockers
B. Beta-adrenergic blockers
C. Potassium channel blockers
D. Calcium channel blockers
E. All of the above

17. All of the following statements concerning propoxyphene are true except

A. Proxyphene is a synthetic opiate agonist
B. Structurally, propoxyphene is more similar to morphine than to methadone
C. Compared with codeine propoxyphene is one half to two thirds as potent an analgesic
D. Propoxyphene exerts little or no antitussive activity

18. Which schedule of drugs listed below would include a drug that is considered to have a strong potential for abuse or addiction but which has legitimate medical use?

A. Schedule I
B. Schedule II
C. Schedule III
D. Schedule IV
E. Schedule V

19. Inhaled ammonia is the drug of choice for acting against
A. Anaphylaxis
B. Heart attack
C. Syncope
D. Urticaria

20. All of the following are useful in the treatment of gout *except*:
A. Allopurinol
B. Aspirin
C. Colchicine
D. Indomethacin
E. Probenecid

21. The major natural mineralocorticoid in humans is:
A. Aldosterone
B. Cortisol
C. Dexamethasone
D. Prednisone

22. Amyl nitrite is used in the emergency treatment of cyanide poisoning because it:
A. Oxidizes hemoglobin
B. Irreversibly binds cyanide
C. Competes with cyanide for binding of cytochromes
D. Inhibits tubular reabsorption of cyanide

23. A pharmacologic antagonist drug:
A. Has no affinity for a receptor and no intrinsic activity
B. Has affinity for a receptor but no intrinsic activity
C. Has affinity for a receptor and intrinsic activity
D. Has no affinity for a receptor but has intrinsic activity

24. When a drug is administered repeatedly, a higher concentration of the drug than is desired may be achieved. The effect of this excessive accumulation is known as:
A. Additive effect
B. Synergistic response
C. Cumulative action
D. Idiosyncrasy

25. The currently available ganglionic blockers for clinical use include:
A. Mecamylamine
B. Hexamethonium
C. Tetraethylammonium
D. Trimethaphan

26. All of the following are phenothiazines except.
A. Chlorpromazine
B. Haloperidol
C. Prochlorperzine
D. Triflupromazine
E. Promazine
F. Trifluoperazine

27. All of the following drugs are used to the treatment of Parkinson's disease *except*.
A. Levodopa
B. Bromocriptine
C. Pergolide
D. Haloperidol
E. Amantadine

28. Methylphenidate is a central nervous system stimulant that is chemically similar to the:
A. Benzodiazepines
B. Amphetamines
C. Phenothiazines
D. Tranquilizers

29. The Controlled Substance act of 1970 uses which criteria listed below for inclusion of a drug into one of the five schedules?
A. Potential for abuse
B. Medical usefulness
C. Degree to which it produces one of physiological dependence
D. Degree to which it produces physical dependence
E. All of the above

30. Which of the following statements are true concerning the occupation theory of drug receptor interaction?

A. It is one of the few theoretical and unifying concepts in pharmacology
B. It follows the law of mass action
C. The theory states that the maximum effects of a drug occurs when all receptors are occupied
D. The theory also states that the magnified of the effect of a drug is proportional to the number of receptors occupied
E. All of the above statements

31. Which of the following drugs can be used in cases of hypotension associated with shock?

A. Prednisone
B. Norepinephrine
C. Pseudoephedrine
D. Lithium

32. Of the following, which is a clinically significant adverse reaction to Cocaine?

A. Epiphyseal closure
B. Hyperkalemia
C. Headache
D. Epistaxis

33. Which of the following are true statements about protein binding?

A. Albumin is the main plasma protein that binds drugs
B. Only bound drugs can interact with receptors to produce therapeutic or toxic effects
C. Drugs can be considered highly protein bound when over 90% of the total drug in plasma is protein-bound.
D. None of the above

34. All of the following statements concerning edrophonium are true except:

A. It is a direct-acting cholinergic agonist (cholinomimetic)
B. It is a rapid-acting, short-duration, parental cholinesterase inhibitor

C. It is the drug of choice for diagnosing myasthenia gravis because of its rapid onset of action and reversibility
D. It is also useful in differentiating a myasthenic crisis from a cholinergic crisis

35. All of the following are macrolide antibiotics except:
A. Erythromycin
B. Azithromycin
C. Clarithromycin
D. Clindamycin

36. Opioid drugs are used therapeutically as all of the following except:
A. Analgesics
B. Antitussives
C. Antiemetics
D. Antidiarrhoeals

37. All of the following drugs are adrenergic agonist except
A. Dopamine
B. Epinephrine
C. Clonidine
D. Phenoxybenzamine
E. Terbutaline
F. Albuterol

38. A contraindication or precaution to the use of propranolol is:
A. Achalasia
B. Renal failure
C. Collagen-vascular disease
D. Near sightedness

39. The most preferable antibiotic for the treatment of a non-penicillinase producing gram positive staphylococcal infection is :
A. Tetracycline
B. Clindamycin
C. Penicillin G or V
D. Ampicillin

40 All of the following drugs are amphetamines except:

A. Benzedrine
B. Dexedrine
C. Morphine
D. Methedrine

41. The penicillinase -resistant drugs are active against aerobes but they are reserved for treating:

A. Candida infections
B. Streptococcal infections
C. Staphylococcal infections
D. Meningococcal infections

42. The brief duration of action of an ultra short acting barbiturate is due to:

A. The slow rate of metabolism in the liver
B. A low lipid solubility, resulting in a minimal concentration in the brain
C. A high degree of binding to plasma proteins
D. A rapid rate of redistribution from the brain due to its high liposolubility
E. A slow rate of excretion by the kidneys

43. All of the following drugs are known to produce orthostatic hypotension as an adverse reaction except:

A. Levodopa
B. Meperidine
C. Chlorpromazine
D. Indomethacin

44. All of the following are optimum alkaloids except

A. Meperidin
B. Morphine
C. Codeine
D. Heroin

45. Which of the following is a contraindication or precaution to the use of Tobramycin

A. Sunlight (UV) exposure
E. Scleroderma

C. Myasthenia gravis
D. Syphilis

46. A therapeutic dose of morphine produces all of the following except.
A. Miosis
B. Decreased GI motility
C. CNS depression
D. Hyperventilation

47. Which antiarrhythmic drug listed below is effective only on the ventricles and is useful in acute ventricular arrhythmias?
A. Quinine
B. Lidocaine
C. Flecainide
D. Propranolol

48. Tetracycline's are the drugs of first choice in the treatment of :
A. Mycoplasma Pneumonia
B. Chlamydia infection
C. Rickettsial infections
D. Vibrio infections
E. All of the above

49. All of the following are components of the typical local anesthetic molecule *except*.
A. An aromatic group
B. A heme group
C. An intermediate chain
D. A secondary or tertiary amino group

50. Buspirone is classified as a (an)
A. Benzodiazepine
B. Azaspirodecanedione
C. Barbiturate
D. Phenothiazine

51. Which of the following is often Co-administered with antibiotics to delay the renal clearance of the antibiotic
A. Aztreonam

B. Imipenem
C. Probenecid
D. Reserpine

52. Alkylating agents are most effective in treating:
A. Chronic leukemias
B. Lymphomas
C. Myelomas
D. Carcinomas of the breast and ovary
E. All of the above

53. All of the following are catecholamines except:
A. Epinephrine
B. Norepinephrine
C. Methyldopa
D. Isoproterenol
E. Dopamine
F. Dobutamine

54. The autonomic nervous system has cholinergic fibers that secrete:
A. Acetylcholine
B. Dopamine
C. Epinephrine
D. Norepinephrine

55. The positive inotropic effect of Digoxin:
A. Is dependent upon a normal cardiac rhythm
B. Directly increases the force of myocardial contractions
C. Is antagonized by beta-blockers
D. All of the above

56. Ethyl alcohol causes a well-marked diuresis by inhibiting the production of:
A. Growth hormone
B. Insulin
C. Antidiuretic hormone (ADH)
D. Epinephrine

57. All of the following are antifungal agents except:
A. Amphotericin B

B. Flucytosine
C. Ketoconazole
D. Polymyxin B
E. Fluconazole
F. Itraconazole

58. All of the following penicillins are acid stable except:
A. Cloxacillin
B. Dicloxacillin
C. Methicillin
D. Nafcillin
E. Oxacillin
F. Pencillin V

59. All of the following are antihistamine H_1 blockers except:
A. Astemizole (Hismanal)
B. Chlorpheniramine (Chlor-Trimeton)
C. Cimetidine
D. Diphenhydramine (Benadryl)
E. Terfenadine (Seldane)

60. Which of the following is most likely to cause cholestasis as an adverse reaction?
A. Ampicillin
B. Diphenhydramine
C. Promethazine
D. Ranitidine

61. Local anesthetics theoretically should be less effective in acutely inflamed tissue than in normal tissue because in inflamed tissue:
A. The pH decreases, thus significantly reducing the concentration of the free-base form of the local anesthetic
B. The pH remains the same, however, the extracellular fluids inactivate the local anesthetic.
C. The pH rises, thus inactivating the anesthetic
D. The pH rises, thus significantly reducing the concentration of the free-base form of the local anesthetic

62. The maximum recommended dose of a local anesthetic that can be administered to a child is determined by:

A. Age
B. Weight
C. Height
D. Gender

63. The dilation of vessels in muscle, the constriction of vessels and a positive inotropic and chronotropic effect on the heart are all action of :

A. Acetylcholine
B. Epinephrine
C. Isoproterenol
D. Metaproterenol

64. Epinephrine reversal is a predictable result of the use of epinephrine in a patient who has received a (an)

A. Beta-blocker
B. Alpha blocker
C. Adrenergic agonist
D. All of the above

65. All of the following statements concerning codeine are true except

A. Codeine is an opiate agonist with chemical structure and effects similar to morphine
B. Codeine is available as phosphate or scuffle salt both of which can be administered by the oral, subcutaneous or intra-muscular route
C. Codeine is much more potent than morphine
D. Codeine is the standard of centrally acting narcotic anti-tussives
E. Codeine has less analgesic respiratory depressive and other side effect than morphine but is a more effective antitussive agent.

66. A teaspoon contains

A. 5 milliliters
B. 10 milliliters

C. 15 milliliters
D. 20 milliliters

67. Tetracycline's should not be used in patient who have
A. Cataracts
B. Leucopenia
C. Severe renal impairment
D. Cardiac disorders

68. Erythromycin is well known to cause adverse :
A. CNS effects
B. GI effects
C. Hematological effects
D. Renal effects

69. All of the following drugs are beta - blockers except
A. Acebutotol
B. Metoprolol
C. Nadolol
D. Prazosin
E. Timolol

70. Adrenaline (epinephrine) stimulates :
A. Alpha 1 receptors
B. Beta 1 receptors
C. Both alpha 1, 2 and beta 1, 2 receptors
D. Alpha 1 and beta 1 receptors only

71. All of the following statements concerning barbiturates are true except.
A. Barbiturates may increase the half lives of drugs metabolized by the liver
B. Barbiturates depress neuronal activity by increasing membrane ion conductance (primarily chloride), reducing glutamate induced depolarization and potentiating the inhibitory effects of GABA
C. Compared with benzondiazepines the barbiturates exhibit a steeper dose response relationship
D. Barbiturates may precipitate acute porphyrias in susceptible patient

72. Of the following penicillin which one has the widest or broadest spectrum of activity?
A. Penicillin G
B. Carbenicillin
C. Oxacillin
D. Cloxacilin

73. Antibiotics administered for angioplasty therapy include
A. Dactinomycin
B. Doxorubicin
C. Bleomycin sulfate
D. Mitomycin
E. All of the above

74. Which of the following species is a catalase positive gram positive bacterium that produces the enzyme beta-lactamase and has been implicated in hospital acquired infections since the 1950's
A. Streptococcus
B. Staphylococcus
C. Mycobacterium
D. Lactobacillus

75. The major clinical use of an opioid antagonist is :
A. In the management of acute alcohol poisoning
B. In the management of status asthmatics
C. In the management of acute opioid overdose
D. In the management of anaphylaxis

76. The term bio-availability of a drug refers to:
A. The movement of a drug into the body tissues over time
B. The dissolution of a drug in the GI tract
C. The measurement of the rate and amount of therapeutic active drug that reaches the systemic circulation
D. The relationship between the physical and chemical properties of a drug and the systemic absorption of the drug
E. The amount of drug destroyed by the liver prior to systemic absorption from GI tract

77. Clindamycin is an antibiotic structurally similar to:
A. Azithromycin
B. Clarithromycin
C. Erythromycin
D. Lincomycin

78. Which of the following are considered to be first-line agents in the treatment of tuberculosis?
A. Isoniazid (INH)
B. Ethambutol
C. Pyrazinamide (PZA)
D. Rifampicin

79. Verapamil is useful for the treatment of :
A. Angina
B. Hypertension
C. Supraventricular tachyarrhythmia
D. All of the above

80. All of the following drugs are monoamine oxidase inhibitors (MAOIs) except
A. Phenelzine
B. Isocarboxazid
C. Imipramine
D. Tranylcypromine

81. Local anesthetics act directly on the membrane by :
A. Increasing K^+ flux
B. Increasing nerve membrane permeability to sodium
C. Decreasing nerve membrane permeability to sodium
D. Increasing membrane excitability

82. The Ester local anesthetics are hydrolyzed primarily in the:
A. Liver
B. Lungs
C. Kidney
D. Plasma

83. An antidiarrheal drug related to meperidine is :
A. Omeprazole
B. Sucralfate

C. Loperamide
D. Metoclopramide

84. The prototype depolarizing neuromuscular blocking agent is:
A. Tubocurarine
B. Mivacurium
C. Vecuronium
D. Succinylcholine
E. Atracurium
F. Rocuronium

85. Biotransformation is also called :
A. Drug elimination
B. Drug Metabolism
C. Drug bioavailability
D. Drug half life

86. The specificity of a drug is most commonly accomplished by altering
A. The solubility
B. The molecular structure
C. The dose
D. The concentration

87. The drug of choice for treating candidiasis is :
A. Chloramphenicol
B. Clindamycin
C. Nystatin
D. Penicillin

88. The antibiotic of choice for prophylactic coverage for the prevention of bacterial endocarditis is:
A. Tetracycline
B. Lincomycin
C. Erythromycin
D. Amoxicillin

89. A vial contains 3.6 ml of a 2% solution of lidocaine with 1:100, 000 epinephrine. How much Lidocaine and epinephrine does this vial contain?

A. 7.2 mg of lidocaine & 0.36 mg of epinephrine
B. 7.2 mg of lidocaine & 0.036 g of epinephrine
C. 72 mg of lidocaine & 0.36 mg of epinephrine
D. 72 mg of lidocaine & 0.036 mg of epinephrine

90. Local anesthetics depress which of the following fibers first?
A. Large myelinated fibers
B. Small unmyelinated fibers
C. Small myelinated fibers
D. Large unmyelinated fibers

91. All of the following statements concerning pilocarpine are true except
A. It is a choline ester
B. It is a direct acting cholinergic agonist (Cholinomimetic)
C. It is lipid soluble
D. The duration of action range from 30 minutes to two hours

92. Which of the following agents has little value in treating acute inflammation
A. Ibuprofen
B. Aspirin
C. Acetaminophen
D. Naproxen

93. The major natural glucocorticoid is:
A. Triamcinolone
B. Cortisol (Hydrocortisone)
C. Dexamethasone (Decadron)
D. Prednisolone (Prelone)

94. All of the following statements concerning Methohexital (Brevital) are true except:
A. It is an ultrashort-acting barbiturate similar to Thiopental
B. It has a faster onset of action and recovery time than does Thiopental
C. It is not as potent as Thiopental
D. It can be used along as an anesthetic for short procedures that are relatively painless, as an inducing agent, or as an adjunct to regional anesthesia

E. Post - anesthesia excitatory phenomena occur more frequently with Methohexital than with Thiopental.

95. Oral contraceptives exert their primary effect by inhibiting:

A. Follicle formation
B. Ovulation
C. Follicle Growth
D. All of the above

96. For a patient who is taking anticoagulants, what is the most valuable test used in evaluating this patient as a surgical risk?

A. PTT (Partial thromboplastin Time)
B. PT (Prothrombin Time)
C. Platelet count
D. Hemoglobin

97. All of the following statements concerning heparin are true except:

A. Heparin inhibits several steps in the intrinsic pathway of blood clotting
B. Heparin is used when anticoagulation is needed immediately
C. It is often used 1 to 2 weeks immediate following a heart attack
D. It passes the placental barrier
E. Increased bleeding is the most common adverse effect of heparin

98. Disulfiram (Antabuse) is used in the management of :

A. Nicotine abuse
B. Ethanol abuse
C. Opioid abuse
D. NSAID abuse

99. Which of the following is a pharmacological antagonist of aldosterone in the collecting tubule?

A. Mannitol
B. Glycerin
C. Isosorbide
D. Urea
E. Spironolactone

100. All of the following are skeletal muscle spasmolytic drugs except
A. Methocarbamol
B. Cyclobenzaprine
C. Baclofen
D. Succinycholine
E. Dantrolene

101. Which of the following has a clinically significant drug interaction with Amoxicillin?
A. Dorzolamide & Timolol
B. Methotrexate
C. Calcitrol
D. Candesartan

102. A drug that acts in a way opposite to the sympathetic nervous system is called a:
A. Sympathomimetic
B. Sympatholytic
C. Sympathetic
D. Adrenergic agent

103. Antipsychotic drugs include:
A. Phenothiazines
B. Thioxanthenes
C. Butyrophenones
D. All of the above

104. All of the following are cholinergic actions except:
A. Slowing of the heart
B. Dilation of the pupils
C. The stimulation of the smooth muscles of the bronchi, GI tract, gallbladder, bile duct, bladder and ureters
D. The stimulation of sweat, salivary, tear and bronchial glands

105. Which agent listed below is used as an antiseptic in mouthwashes and skin wound cleansers?
A. Dexamethasone
B. Hexylresorcinol
C. Epinephrine
D. Penicillin

106. All of the following drugs are alpha blockers except:

A. Doxazosin
B. Phenoxybenzamine hydrochloride
C. Phentolamine hydrochloride
D. Propranolol
E. Terazosin

107. Nitroglycerin either directly or through reflexes result in all of the following except:

A. Increased heart rate
B. Increased venous capacity
C. Decreased cardiac force
D. Decreased after-load

108. Aluminum salt used as antacids include:

A. Hydroxide
B. Carbonate
C. Phosphate
D. Amino acetate
E. All of the above

109. Pain that has no organic basis and is fixed upon some portion of the anatomy is referred to as:

A. Intractable pain
B. Referred pain
C. Psychogenic pain
D. Phantom pain

110. All of the following are effects of insulin except:

A. Decreased gluconeogenesis
B. Increased triglyceride storage
C. Decreased protein synthesis
D. Increased glycogen synthesis

111. Tissue thromboplastin is considered to be coagulation factor

A. I
B. II
C. III
D. IV

112. Prominent toxic effects of mercury include all of the following except

A. Acute renal failure
B. Tremors
C. Salivation
D. Mydriasis
E. Slurred speech
F. Loosened teeth

113. All of the following are angiotensin - converting enzyme (ACE) inhibitors except

A. Captopril
B. Hydralazine
C. Enalapril
D. Lisnopril

114. If norepinephrine or epinephrine were to stimulate or combine with the alpha - receptors in the eye, which response listed below would you except?

A. Miosis (Contraction of the pupil)
B. Mydriasis (dilation of the pupil)
C. Neither of the above; nor - epinephrine and epinephrine do not stimulate or combine with alpha receptors in the eye

115. Which antibiotic listed below is used cautiously due to its side effects pseudomembranous colitis (severe GI upset)?

A. Clindamycin
B. Cloxacillin
C. Erythromycin
D. Vancomycin

116. Which of the following side effects are most common with the use of Diazepam (Valium)?

A. Rash, itch
B. Mouth, throat ulcers
C. Drowsiness, fatigue
D. Difficulty with urination

117. Which of the following is a contraindication or precaution to the use of Cefotaxime?

A. Scoliosis

B. Bronchitis
C. Aortic Stenosis
D. Breast-feeding

118. The amide local anesthetics are metabolized primarily in the:
A. Lungs
B. Plasma
C. Liver
D. Kidney

119. All of the following are benzodiazepines except
A. Lorazapam
B. Oxazepam
C. Alprazolam
D. Carbamazepine
E. Midazolam

120. Ethosuximide is effective in treating absence seizures by causing
A. Sodium channel blockade
B. Neuronal membrane hyperpolarization
C. Calcium channel blockade
D. GABA-chloride channel blockade

121. Sulfonamides are structurally similar to :
A. Penicillin
B. PABA (para aminobenzoic acid)
C. Salicylic acid
D. Ergotamine

122. Which alpha - adrenergic blocker listed below is used for persistent pulmonary hypertension of the newborn and for treating peripheral vasoplastic disorders in adults
A. Prazosin
B. Terazosin
C. Tolazolin
D. Doxazosin
E. Phentolamine
F. Phenoxybenzamine (dibenzylene)

123. Local anaesthetics

A. Greatly decreases the resting potential of peripheral nerves
B. Act on the extracellular surface of the nerve membrane in the uncharged state
C. Prevent the development of the action potential of a nerve
D. Block nerve conduction by interfering with calcium conductance

124. A drug with a high LD_{50} and a Ed_{50} has a

A. High therapeutic index and is therefore very dangerous
B. High therapeutic index and is therefore relativity safe
C. Low therapeutic index and is therefore very dangerous
D. Low therapeutic index and is therefore relativity safe

125. All of the following drugs are cardiac glycosides (cardio - tonics) except:

A. Amrinone
B. Deslanoside
C. Digoxin
D. Propranolol
E. Digitoxin
F. Ouabain

126. Which term listed bellows is a compulsive, uncontrollable dependence on a substance, habit or practice to such a degree that cessation causes severe emotional mental or physiological reactions?

A. Habituation
B. Tolerance
C. Addiction
D. None of the above

127. An international Unit of a substance is:

A. The amount that is eliminated by the kidneys
B. The amount that produces a specific biological result
C. The amount that produces toxicity
D. The amount that is bound to protein

128. Acyclovir can be used to treat

A. Tuberculosis
B. Varicella - zoster virus infections

C. Atrial fibrillation
D. Anticholinergic syndrome

129. The body contains three types of endogenous opioids which one of the following is not one of them?
A. Beta-endorphins
B. Morphine
C. Enkephalins
D. Dynorphins

130. All of the following fibers are cholinergic except
A. Preganglionic sympathetic fibers
B. Preganglionic parasympathetic fibers
C. Postganglionic sympathetic fibers
D. Postganglionic parasympathetic fibers

131. Which from of a local anesthetic can readily penetrate tissue membrane?
A. Ionized form
B. Non-ionized free base form
C. Ionized and non-ionized form
D. None of the above

132. Which of the following presents the greatest danger of penicillin therapy?
A. GI upset
B. CNS irritation
C. An allergic reaction
D. Renal damage

133. Alpha receptors are located on:
A. Vascular smooth muscle
B. Presynaptic nerve terminals
C. Blood platelets
D. Fat cells
E. Neurons in the CNS
F. All of the above

134. All of the following statements concerning toxicity are true except
A. Toxicity is often an extension of the desired drug effect

B. Toxicity is dose dependent but not time dependent
C. Toxicity can be anything ranging from nausea to death
D. Toxicity can be caused by even minimal concentrations of a drug

135. Acetazolamide is a:
A. Loop diuretic
B. Carbonic anhydrase inhibitor
C. Thiazide diuretic
D. Potassium sparing diuretic

136. All of the following are choline esters except:
A. Pilocarpine
B. Methacholine
C. Bethanechol
D. Carbachol

137. For which of the following conditions can ranitidine be used?
A. Prostatitis
B. Pyrosis (heart burn)
C. Toxic-shock syndrome
D. Renal failure

138. Cephalosporins have which of the following mode of action?
A. Affect cell membrane
B. Interfere with protein synthesis
C. Affect cell wall
D. Interfere with normal biosynthetic pathways

139. Which insulin zinc suspension listed below has the longest duration of action
A. Ultra-lente insulin
B. Semilente insulin
C. Lente insulin
D. None of the above

140. The treatment of the pseudomembranous colitis caused by clindamycin is
A. Penicillin
B. Streptomycin
C. Tetracycline
D. Vancomycin

141. All of the following are CNS stimulants except:
A. Pentylenetetrazol
B. Doxapram
C. Phenobarbital
D. Nikethamide
E. Picrotoxin
F. Strychnine

142. The heart is generally considered to have predominantly which type of adrenergic receptors
A. Alpha 1
B. Alpha 2
C. Beta 1
D. Beta 2

143. All of the following drugs are neuronal blockers except:
A. Guanethidine
B. Guanadrel
C. Clonidine
D. Reserpine

144. The prototype penicillin is :
A. Penicillin V
B. Penicillin G
C. Ampicillin
D. Nafcillin

145. Clinically, Scopolamine is used to:
A. Prevent motion sickness
B. Reduces salivation and excess bronchial secretion prior to surgery
C. Reduces spastic states in Parkinsonism
D. Treat iritis and uveitis
E. All of the above

146. Of the following which is a clinically significant adverse reaction due to Diphenhydramine (Benadryl)?
A. Hypovitaminosis
B. Paresthesia
C. Contact dermatitis
D. Delirium

147. All of the following are anti - HIV agents except:

A. Didanosine
B. Ganciclovir
C. Ritonavir
D. Lamivudine
E. Indinavir

148. The maximal recommended adult dose of Lidocaine is 300 mg. How many milliliters of 2% Lidocaine need to be given to reach this level?

A. 7.5 milliliters
B. 10 milliliters
C. 15 milliliters
D. 20 milliliters

149. Lithium is the drug of choice in treating:

A. Unipolar disorders
B. Bipolar affective disorder
C. Migraines
D. Pain

150. All of the following contain aspirin except:

A. Darvon Compound-65
B. Fiorinal
C. Tylenol
D. Empirin with Codeine # 3 or # 4
E. Diflunisal

151. Which of the following are broncho-dilators:

A. Theophylline
B. Aminophylline
C. Epinephrine
D. Terbutaline
E. Albuterol
F. All of the above.

152. All of the following statements concerning ibuprofen are true except:

A. It has a half-life of about 2 hours
B. It is relatively safe

C. It produces more GI disturbances than does aspirin
D. It is well absorbed after oral administration and is excreted via the kidney
E. It is the least expensive of the newer NSAID's (Naproxen, Indomethacin, etc.)
F. It is available in low-dose over the counter formulations

153. All of the following are cholinesterase inhibitors except:
A. Physostigmine
B. Neostigmine
C. Edrophonium
D. Methacholine
E. Pyridostigmine

154. The physiochemical properties of drugs that influence their passage across biologic membranes are:
A. Lipid solubility
B. Degree of ionization
C. Molecular size and shape
D. All of the above

155. The major disadvantages with the use of opioid analgesics is:
A. Allergic response
B. Nausea
C. Vomiting
D. Respiratory depression

156. Growth hormone is also called:
A. Vasopressin
B. Aldosterone
C. Somatotropin
D. Dopamine

157. Antimetabolites are cell cycle-specific drugs, acting primarily in the:
A. G 0 phase or resting phase of the cell cycle
B. S phase of the cell cycle
C. G 1 phase of the cell cycle
D. G 2 phase of the cell cycle

158. Which route of drug administration listed below will give the most rapid onset of pharmacological effect?

A. Oral administration
B. Subcutaneous injection
C. Intravenous injection
D. Intramuscular injection

159. All of the following are pharmacologic effects of glucocorticoids except:

A. A decrease in gluconeogenesis
B. A decrease in the utilization of glucose
C. The inhibition of protein synthesis
D. An increase in protein catabolism
E. A decreased resistance to infection

160. Which route of administration of a drug listed below is most known for its significant hepatic "first pass" metabolism?

A. Intramuscular
B. Inhalation
C. Sublingual
D. Oral

161. All of the following sites are generally accepted for IM injections except:

A. The buttocks
B. The biceps muscle
C. The deltoid muscle
D. The anterior thigh

162. Quinacrine is an oral anti-protozoal agent used most commonly in the treatment of:

A. Chronic bronchitis
B. AIDS
C. Giardiasis
D. Leprosy

163. The only nonbarbiturate sedative-hypnotic agent that is indicated in the practice of dentistry is:

A. Pentobarbital
B. Secobarbital

C. Chloral hydrate
D. Meperidine

164. Which of the following is a contraindication or precaution to the use of Procainamide?
A. Polycystic ovary syndrome
B. Ester local anesthetic hypersensitivity
C. Thrombocytopenia
D. Acute myocardial infarction

165. Which of the following is a pharmacologic antagonist of aldosterone in the collecting tubule?
A. Mannitol
B. Glycerin
C. Spironolactone
D. Isosorbide
E. Urea

166. All of the following are skeletal muscle spasmolytic drugs except:
A. Methocarbamol
B. Cyclobenzaprine
C. Baclofen
D. Succinylcholine
E. Dantrolene

167. All of the following drugs are indirect-acting adrenergic agonists except:
A. Tyramine
B. Amphetamine
C. Epinephrine
D. Methamphetamine
E. Hydroxyamphetamine

168. The safest and easiest route for drug administration is:
A. Oral
B. IV
C. Rectal
D. Inhalation

169. Which of the following routes of drug administration is generally used for local drug effects?

A. Topical administration
B. Oral ingestion
C. Subcutaneous injection
D. Intravenous injection

170. Which of the following refers to the efficacy of a drug?

A. The relative concentrations of two or more drugs that produce the same drug effect
B. The ability of a drug to produce a desired therapeutic effect regardless of dosage
C. The dose of a drug that will kill a patient
D. None of the above

Answer Key to MCQs in Pharmacology

1	D	2	ACFG	3	C	4	C
5	A	6	D	7	D	8	C
9	C	10	D	11	C	12	I
13	C	14	A	15	E	16	E
17	B	18	B	19	C	20	B
21	A	22	A	23	B	24	C
25	A,D	26	B	27	D	28	B
29	E	30	E	31	B	32	C
33	A, C	34	A	35	D	36	C
37	D	38	B	39	C	40	C
41	C	42	D	43	D	44	A
45	C	46	D	47	B	48	E
49	B	50	B	51	C	52	E
53	C	54	A	55	B	56	C
57	D	58	C	59	C	60	C
61	A	62	B	63	B	64	B
65	C	66	A	67	C	68	B
69	D	70	C	71	A	72	B
73	E	74	B	75	C	76	C
77	D	78	A, D	79	D	80	C

81	C	82	D	83	C	84	D
85	B	86	B	87	C	88	D
89	D	90	B	91	A	92	C
93	B	94	C	95	B	96	B
97	D	98	B	99	E	100	D
101	B	102	B	103	D	104	B
105	B	106	D	107	C	108	E
109	D	110	C	111	C	112	D
113	B	114	B	115	A	116	C
117	D	118	C	119	D	120	C
121	B	122	C	123	C	124	B
125	D	126	C	127	B	128	B
129	B	130	C	131	B	132	C
133	F	134	B	135	B	136	A
137	B	138	C	139	A	140	D
141	C	142	C	143	C	144	B
145	E	146	C	147	B	148	C
149	B	150	C	151	F	152	C
153	D	154	D	155	D	156	C
157	B	158	C	159	A	160	D
161	B	162	C	163	C	164	B
165	C	166	D	167	C	168	A
169	A	170	B				

Reader's Notes

Reader's Notes